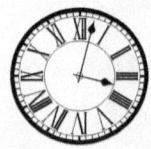

MALIK PUBLISHING GROUP

An Imprint of Malik Ventures Group

New York, NY

Copyright © 2022 by Param Malik

All rights reserved, including rights to reproduce this book in its entirety or portions thereof in any form. No portion of this book may be used or reproduced without the explicit written permission of the author, except in the case where brief quotation is necessary for articles and reviews. All inquiries must be addressed to the author directly.

Malik Publishing Group (MPG) and colophon are the intellectual property of Malik Ventures Group (MVG)

Title: *Exploring Life: Probing Human Life, Disease, & the Landscape of Modern Medicine*

Printed in the United States of America

ISBN: 9798849296470

10 8 6 4 2 1 3 5 7 9

EXPLORING LIFE

PROBING HUMAN LIFE, DISEASE, & THE
LANDSCAPE OF MODERN MEDICINE

EXPLORING LIFE

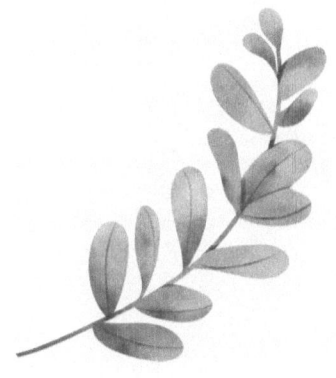

PROBING HUMAN LIFE, DISEASE, & THE LANDSCAPE OF MODERN MEDICINE

PARAM MALIK

*To all who have believed in me,
to all who have touched my life,
and to all whose wisdom has enlightened me.....*

CONTENTS

INTRODUCTION	1
CHAOS THE FABRIC OF LIFE	7
GENOME	27
FACETS OF OUR PHYSIOLOGY	43
RHYTHM	73
IMMUNITY THE STEWARD OF OUR WELL-BEING	85
MALADY	97
ELIXIR	121
AUTHOR'S NOTE ACKNOWLEDGEMENTS SELECTED BIBLIOGRAPHY EXPANDED GLOSSARY	155

EXPANDED CONTENTS

INTRODUCTION | 1

CHAOS | 7
MOLECULES OF THE CELL
RESPIRATION OF THE CELL
COMMUNICATION OF THE CELL
VITAMINS & MINERALS

GENOME | 27
DISCOVERING THE GENOME
DECIPHERING THE GENOME
DISCERNING THE GENOME

FACETS | 43
OUR MICROBIOME
DIGESTION
BREATHING
CIRCULATION
ENDOCRINOLOGY - OUR HORMONES
NEUROPHYSIOLOGY
SENSATION & MOVEMENT
RENAL PHYSIOLOGY
HOMEOSTASIS

EXPANDED CONTENTS

RHYTHMS | 73
THE CIRCADIAN CLOCK
SLEEP
DREAMING
CAFFEINE & SLEEP
SLEEP DEPRIVATION

IMMUNITY | 85
IMMUNITY

MALADY | 97
AGING & SENESCENCE
CANCER
AUTOIMMUNITY
NEURODEGENERATION
DIABETES
ARTHRITIS
ASTHMA
GENETIC DISORDERS
ACUTE DISEASES & INFECTIONS
CARDIOVASCULAR DISEASE
STROKE

EXPANDED CONTENTS

ELIXIR | 121
ALTERNATIVE MEDICINE
AYURVEDA
PHARMACOLOGY
MODEL ORGANISMS IN RESEARCH
SURGERY
ANESTHETICS
ANTIBIOTICS & ANTIVIRALS
VACCINES
STEM CELL THERAPY
GENETIC ENGINEERING
CRISPR
AGING RESEARCH
CHEMOTHERAPY & TARGETED THERAPY
IMMUNOTHERAPY

AUTHOR'S NOTE | 155
ACKNOWLEDGEMENTS
ABOUT THE AUTHOR
SELECTED BIBLIOGRAPHY
EXPANDED GLOSSARY

EXPLORING LIFE

PROBING HUMAN LIFE, DISEASE, & THE
LANDSCAPE OF MODERN MEDICINE

INTRODUCTION

"If chemistry was the science of the nineteenth century, and physics the science of the twentieth, then surely, biomedicine must be the science of the twenty-first century..."

- Dr. Lloyd B. Minor

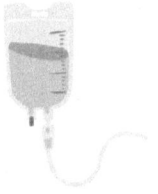

    Our understanding of the evolution, flourishing, and continuity of the human species is fundamental to our approach in setting forth the advances that will shape modern-day medicine. Our study of the biology of natural systems, the very processes that keep us conscious and alive, offers us a broadened perspective on life. Our modern species has been shaped by survival of the fittest-

a kind of natural selection. Our species has also been shaped by disease and healing - the reciprocity between malady and elixir. The practice of medicine emerged as the craft of healing long before any fundamental understanding of human biology. The medical field, however, with its numerous present-day branches, has since evolved into a practice that underlies its foundations in a fundamental understanding of human biology. For it is only with the greatest understanding of our fundamental biological processes - the most intricate facets of our physiology - that we can fully grasp the magnitude of a disease and innovate a better path to a cure. Our doctors and scientists - the sages and savants of our day - are pushing the modern-day practice of healthcare into newer boundaries.

Malady has stepped into every facet of our lives; disease is an integral part of our existence, a kind of dual-citizenship. What is the purpose of life if we are all to be ill? What is the essence of existence when nature has devised schemes to contest it? What are the mechanisms behind disease, we may ask. What triggers the tumor? How does the body succumb to illness? Fundamental questions like these pervade our urgent need for answers. It has been, once again, our understanding of biology that has offered us the most meaningful explanations to our most urgent questions.

In this engrossing narrative of the field, we explore what has transformed biomedicine into the greatest disci-

-pline of our epoch, and delve into the most fulfilling explanations to some of our most expansive questions. We will explore our body from the genes in our nucleus to the neurotransmitters in our brains. We will explore how inhibition, suppression, and elicitation have been the commonality between many of our largest medical breakthroughs. We will explore the most fundamental advances made in medicine in the midst of scientific abstraction. We will explore the questions that are yet to be answered by science.

This book is written for all with a curious mind. It is for all who want to understand life and nature, all who want to learn about the practice of medicine, and for all who want to understand how our study of living systems has transformed our capacity to treat illness and expanded the offerings of medical care. It is for all who want to understand how biology has transformed the practice of medicine, for it has been the deft understanding of our past that has allowed us to make the greatest of strides for our species. It has been our understanding of biology, in essence, that has transformed the practice of medicine.

As you read this book, I urge you to make connections between phenomena and to think abstractly. I ask you to consider your own existence and the composition of your own physiology, and recognize the highly intricate yet elegant processes that make you who you are. Your -

physiology is a work to be celebrated. Recognize the efforts of your trillions of cells, each with nearly 23 trillion molecules, and billions of chemical reactions occurring at any given moment. Acknowledge your existence as the result of 3.8 billion years of evolution from the simplest prokaryote to the complex being that you are. In many ways, you will be able to discover yourself - your inner self. You will, of course, learn about the discoveries of hundreds of scientists, physicians, anatomists, and physiologists. You may be inspired to study a topic further, and I encourage you to take that step in your education.

You will also learn about disease. Nature has kept a particularly keen class of adversaries dangerously close to us, hovering over our lives, and for some of us, affecting almost every second of our day. Whether you finish *Malady* with a newfound familiarity of numerous diseases and disorders, or have understood a little better the mechanisms behind your particular cancer or genetic syndrome, you will certainly find solace and consolation after reading *Elixir,* upon learning about the wealth of advancements and therapies that have flooded our hospitals and offered patients newfound confidence in the modern-day practice of medicine. While there is still much work needed in the field, incredible progress has been made, and incurable diseases that had previously shaken populations are now treatable.

INTRODUCTION

I've written this book as an attempted account of the remarkable intricacies of human biology and the outstanding discoveries that have helped shape the medical field. This book is neither a textbook nor a story, it is instead a narrative of the biomedical field that attempts to encapsulate the greatest of strides in science and medicine. It's crucial to note that, in the interest of keeping this book to a reasonable length that will appeal to a wide range of readers, an in-depth coverage of certain topics and diseases has been excluded from this book. I try my best to convey sympathy when discussing about the prognostic intricacies of certain diseases. Even so, please note that much of the discussions of such topics are kept more *informative* than *narrative*, and due to the limitations of space in this book, I am unable to provide as much sympathy in these cases as I would have liked. I ask you to keep this in mind as you approach the pages in *Malady*.

Generation after generation, we have increasingly prioritized the study of science and the practice of medicine. It has been this unwavering focus that has brought us meaningful innovation in healthcare. Science has brought the most meaningful advances in our lives, and our understanding of biology has shaped our approach to medicine. The steadfast commitment to learning about our most intricate processes has yielded the greatest breakthroughs in human health, and will continue to do so for as long as we make the practice of research and discovery a multigenerational priority. As we will observe throughout this book, biology has, and will continue to, shape the practice of medicine.

CHAOS

PART ONE:

CHAOS

THE FABRIC OF LIFE

"Life is not found in atoms or molecules as such, but in organization; not in symbiosis, but in synthesis..."

- E. Grant Conklin

The study of our biology and the field of medicine begins with an understanding of our most fundamental biochemical interactions: *biochemistry* in its most elaborate sense.

—

Until now, you may simply know that our body is composed of organs, and our organs are composed of tissues. You may have known tissues are groups of cells, and cells are the fundamental unit of life. And you may know our cells are made of biological molecules. Let's understand the *molecules* of the cell.

Molecules of the Cell

To understand the interactions within molecules is to fathom a world of great chaos, disorder, and spontaneity. The atomic world completely contradicts rationale, order, and purpose. Take two atoms, whose path to collision and bonding is so wild and spontaneous that we wonder how our much larger organ structures and the world around us maintain shape - how our anatomy is intact, when the very pillars of our construct move and collide so unpredictably. The quantum level is one that contradicts much of our understanding of physics, mathematics, and nature. It is instead a level of probability and chance.

From this infinitesimal world of chaos and disorder arises structure, synchrony, and rhythm. These spontaneous bonds between atoms are the foundations of our four most essential biological molecules: carbohydrates, proteins, nucleic acids, and lipids. When we transition from the level of the atom to that of the molecule, order and organization are more apparent. It is a domain where structure determines function. Whether it be the binding of an enzyme to its substrate, or an antibody recognizing the antigen on the surface of a cell, every molecule in biology is designed with its purpose in mind.

Consider for a moment why our bodies require food. Our cells need to produce Adenosine Triphosphate (ATP), a type of energy currency of the cell. Our cells use ATP to drive many processes, including nerve impulse propagation, muscle contraction, synthesis of biochemicals and molecules, and intracellular signaling. ATP is produced in our cells through a complex process known as cellular respiration, where carbohydrates and oxygen molecules are broken down and converted into carbon dioxide and approximately 30-32 molecules of ATP are produced (total yield per glucose molecule). In fact, the reason why we need to consume glucose in our diet is that our cells require it for ATP production, and our bodies are unable to make glucose for ourselves in the way plants can.

While glucose is used in aerobic cellular respiration, it is only one of many carbohydrates existing in living systems. Cellulose, a linked chain of thousands of glucose units, is used by plant cells in providing structure to the rigid cell wall. Starch is a polysaccharide that stores energy for plants. Lactose, a disaccharide, is a sugar found in milk products and consists of galactose molecules with glucose subunits.

Enzymes are one type of a much more diverse set of biological molecules known as proteins. Proteins, known for facilitating a vast array of functions including catalyzing metabolic reactions (enzymes), providing structure to cells (structural proteins), transporting molecules (transport proteins), responding to stimuli, -

---

* If it helps, when you hear a molecule ending in -ose, think "sugar". Likewise, when you hear a molecule ending in -ase, think of "enzyme".

(signaling proteins), and relaying chemical signals (hormones), are involved in practically every process within living cells.

Before we continue exploring other biological molecules central to the activities of the cell, let's first delve into the origins of biochemistry and a crucial metabolic process of the cell.

Respiration of Cells

The first half of the twentieth century saw the emergence of molecular biology and biochemistry as entirely new disciplines, largely initiated by German physiologist Eduard Buchner's experiment of cell-free alcoholic fermentation. While Buchner refined new techniques for breaking yeast cells without damaging the organelles inside, he inspired a much more significant movement - breaking down the chemical stages of complex biological processes.

Continuing on the discoveries of the processes of respiration and fermentation, German physician Otto Meyerhof studied the production of lactic acid through the breakdown of stored glycogen. His work underlies an important metabolic principle: when oxygen is not available, our cells convert glucose to energy using fats, a process known as *fermentation*. Lactic acid is the byproduct of that process. This is often observed when we, for instance, run too fast to catch our breath (and obtain enough oxygen), and our muscles feel sore. This -

"soreness" is actually the buildup of lactic acid, proof that our body has adapted to hypoxic conditions and started to metabolize our excess fat reserves for energy.

Karl Lohmann, a witty student of Meyerhof, characterized ATP as what we consider to be the energy currency of the cell. ATP is the product of cellular respiration, the result of metabolizing glucose molecules. Later, we will explore how ATP is actually used throughout the body. But for now, it's important to note that ATP is the energy currency of the cell - it is the herald that powers the most fundamental aspects of our physiology.

Another scientist, by the name of Otto Warburg, purified and characterized the enzymes involved in the intricate process of cellular respiration. His "Warburg apparatus" allowed for precise measurements of the gases released and consumed throughout the duration of the reactions of cellular respiration. He also used a spectrophotometer to detect the absorption of light by the molecules involved.

Most notably, Warburg discovered that cancer cells undergo fermentation (a process typically reserved for when oxygen is not available) in the presence of oxygen. We will explore this phenomenon further in *Malady*.

Hans Krebs, a student of Warburg, discovered that certain metabolic transformations corresponded to a cyc-

-lical set of reactions. This cyclical series of reactions was termed the "Krebs Cycle", alternatively referred to as the "Citric Acid Cycle".

Putting this newfound knowledge together, along with many other discoveries offering insights novel insights into the intricate mechanisms of metabolism, we now are able to delve into one of the most elegant and refined, and yet one the most profound affairs of the cell.

Cellular respiration begins with a molecule of glucose entering the cell. Once in the cytoplasm, a group of enzymes (including Hexokinase, several isomerases, aldolases, dehydrogenases, and finally pyruvate kinase) gradually convert this glucose molecule into pyruvate (pyruvic acid).

Before we explore the next step in this process, we must first familiarize ourselves with a particularly adept molecule called *Nicotinamide Adenine Dinucleotide*, or *NAD*. Note that when a NAD molecule is *chemically oxidized*, it loses an electron, and is referred to as NAD+. When NAD is *chemically reduced*, it gains an electron, and is referred to as NADH (H for hydrogen). NAD is often involved in carrying electrons from one molecular reaction to another, almost like an electron transporter. In addition to facilitating the transfer of electrons between reactions, however, NAD is secondly used as a substrate of enzymes responsible for adding or removing chemical groups or side chains to, or from, proteins in posttranslational modifications. Keep your recollection of the NAD molecule; we may delve into its interesting relationships with aging in *Malady*.

The pyruvate molecule is then decarboxylated (oxidized and carboxyl group is removed) into an acetyl-coenzyme A (acetyl-CoA). This reaction generates carbon dioxide (CO_2) as a byproduct. CO_2 is subsequently transported through the systemic veins or pulmonary arteries to the lungs where it is exhaled.

This acetyl-CoA molecule enters the matrix of the mitochondrion of the cell, where it is greeted by a truculent rush of metabolic enzymes primed to rearrange its molecular structure and generate from it yet another twenty molecules of ATP, six molecules of NADH, and 2 molecules of $FADH_2$ through the Krebs Cycle.

The final process of aerobic cellular respiration – *oxidative phosphorylation* – occurs in the cristae (inner membrane) of the mitochondrion. Oxygen acts as the final electron acceptor, waiting at the end of a decorous electron transport chain to grab an electron (as it often does).

The outcome of this elaborate process – the result of aerobic cellular respiration – is enough molecules of ATP to meet the energy demands of the cell (30 to 32 ATP molecules per molecule of glucose, to be exact).

Why is *ATP (Adenosine 5'-Triphosphate)* the preferred currency of energy for the cell, you may ask, especially when considering that *GTP* is used many times for similar purposes? Why is it the primary molecule for storing and transferring energy in our cells? ATP is, in fact, an excellent molecule for storing energy, due to the phosphate groups that link through the phosphodiester bonds within the molecule.

Like our deposit of dollars in a bank, ATP can be used to store energy for future reactions or be withdrawn when energy for reactions in the cell is needed. ATP is a nucleic acid, consisting of an adenine base attached to a ribose sugar. In ATP, that sugar is attached to three phosphate groups, hence the term *triphosphate*. When ATP is converted to ADP (Adenosine Diphosphate) or AMP (Adenosine Monophosphate), it now has two or one remaining phosphate group. This *dephosphorylation* represents the release of energy stored in ATP. In the cell, ATP, ADP, and AMP are constantly interconverted in biochemical reactions.

Certain reactions in the cell are not favorable and will not inherently occur. Following input of energy, these reactions become favorable for the cell. These reactions require the phosphorylation or dephosphorylation of ATP.

We have until now reserved a discussion on the different uses of ATP in the cell. This is because in order to und-

-erstand ATP's work in the cell, and its remarkable contributions to the cellular environment, we needed to first understand ATP's origin story - how it's synthesized and how it's evolved to represent the energy currency of the cell.

The uses of ATP in the body are vast. Firstly, ATP is heavily involved with the transduction of cellular signals by serving as a substrate for the kinase enzyme. Note that enzymes are responsible for catalyzing biological reactions by converting its substrates into products. Nearly every metabolic process in the cell (and of course, in the body) requires enzyme catalysis to occur in order to facilitate the metabolic reaction at a rate fast enough to sustain life. We currently know over 5,000 types of biochemical reactions that utilize enzymes.

ATP is one of four molecules involved in the synthesis of RNA, a major genetic molecule of the cell, and the replication and transcription of DNA require the consumption of ATP.

Further, ATP is used in the production of proteins, transporting chemicals out of or into a cell against a concentration gradient, and at times acts as a signal to communicate with other cells regarding particular physiological information. In fact, ATP serves as a neurotransmitter as well, sending signals across the brain and between neurons.

Nucleic Acids

As the bonds between the base, sugar, and phosphate in nucleotides were being deciphered, the distinctions between DNA and RNA became more apparent. Various individuals had proposed that DNA was the molecule of the animal world, and RNA that of the world of plants. Others understood DNA as a continuous repetition of four nucleotide bases. With this introduction, let's delve into nucleic acids, another type of biological macromolecule.

Nucleic acids are large biological molecules that contain the blueprint for life. Two large forms include deoxyribonucleic acids (DNA) and ribonucleic acids (RNA). DNA is a double-stranded molecule, and carries the genetic information for the development and functioning of many organisms, including humans. We will further explore nucleic acids and DNA in Genome.

RNA is a single-stranded molecule that, in humans, is used to transfer genetic information from DNA to proteins, during the translation stage of gene expression. Several other organisms, including particular viruses and microbes, use RNA instead of DNA as the primary genetic molecule of the cell. In fact, RNA is widely regarded to be the first genetic molecule to arise in biological organisms, where a primitive form evolved into the RNA and DNA found in organisms today.

Communication of the Cell

The survival of any cell depends on its reception and processing of various extracellular signals. Whether it be pertaining to the availability of nutrients, directions for producing a protein, or growth factors, our cells have evolved a variety of signaling mechanisms to accomplish the transmission of essential biological information. It is for this reason that the cellular microenvironment is as intricate and complex as the cell itself.

—

For any cell to respond to environmental alterations, it must be capable of receiving, processing, and responding to extracellular signals. While individual cells often receive many signal simultaneously, the information is often integrated into a single plan of action for the cell.

The signals that cells receive are mostly chemical in nature. Where prokaryotes carry sensors that, upon detection of nutrients, navigate the cell toward nutrient sources, multicellular organisms utilize growth factors, hormones, neurotransmitters, and components of the extracellular matrix. Some of these substanes may exert effects locally or might travel to distant cells. Neurotransmitters travel relatively small distances across the space between neurons. Many hormones, however, may travel across entire organs to reach a target.

Each cell contains millions of receptors on its surface. These receptors bind to signaling molecules and initiate a physiological response. Receptors are typically transmembrane proteins, and bind to signaling molecules extracellularly, resulting in a subsequent transmission of the signal through a sequence of molecular events referred to as a signal transduction cascade.

Through such cascades, the signal is typically amplified within the cell and results in the expression of a particular gene and the subsequent formation of a particular protein product.

Types of Cell Signaling Receptors

Ion-Gated Channels

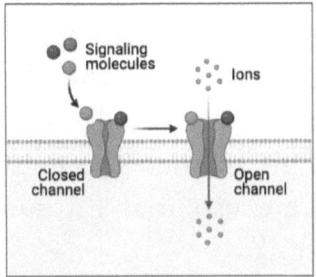

Enzyme-Linked

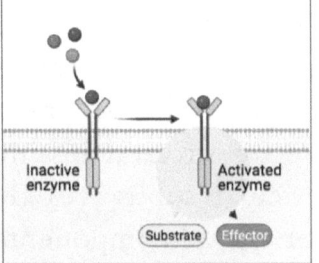

G-Protein Coupled Receptors

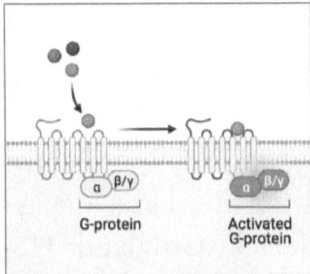

Intracellular Signaling

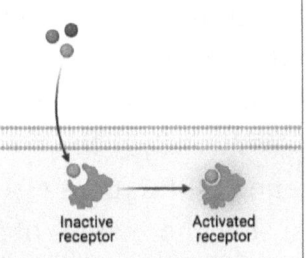

Vitamins & Minerals

A more pronounced class of molecules, whose discovery helped enhance the visibility of biochemistry and convinced the world of its great usefulness, is that of vitamins.

A widespread understanding of deficiency diseases had emerged in the 1880s - diseases resulting from the lack of an essential substance in the body. Several scientists had discovered that, whereas milk has a complete "food" for the body, a diet consisting solely of the known components of milk, rather than milk itself, was not suitable for survival in mice. This implied the existence of particular substances that were essential for survival and not typical components of milk.

In 1912, Polish biochemist Casimir Funk coined the term "vitamin" to describe the active element that he believed he had extracted that had prevented the onset of beriberi in an experiment. The term was derived from "vita" - meaning life - and "amine" - referring to nitrogenous substances essential for life. Later that year, a chemist by the name of Frederick Gowland Hopkins defined vitamins more generally as elements essential in the diet (in very small quantities). In the years following, Hopkins and his colleagues isolated and purified various other vitamins, and explained the reason behind vitamins' necessity in the diet. He characterized vitamins as coenzymes - smaller molecules essential to the primary action of the enzyme.

In fact, the precise requirements of vitamins by our body have been a matter of debate for nearly two centuries. Scientists began to observe that certain diseases and disorders were in fact the result of vitamin deficiencies.

Further, certain vitamins are fat-soluble (dissolve in adipose tissues, *hydrophobic*) and typically accumulate in the body. These include Vitamin A, Vitamin D, Vitamin E, and Vitamin K. However, other vitamins are only water-soluble (hydrophilic), and cannot be stored in the body. Unused water-soluble vitamins are typically excreted out of the body. This is why our bodies require constant consumption of Vitamin C and the Vitamin B complex (i.e. B6, B12).

To highlight a few notable vitamins, Vitamin A helps in immunity and vision, and restores the health and function of the skin and surface linings of our body. The Vitamin B complex helps in the release of energy from the food we consume, as well as in maintaining the health of the nervous system. Vitamin C helps in fighting infection and healing of wounds. Vitamin D helps our body absorb calcium, indirectly restoring bone health. Vitamin E helps maintain cell structure, including the cell membrane, and Vitamin K helps with blood clotting.*

---

* Only the generic functions of vitamins A, B, C, D, and E have been included as these vitamins are relatively notable. For a more thorough list of vitamins and functions, I would direct you to the following articles and vitamin/mineral databases by the National Institute of Health:

- https://www.nia.nih.gov/health/vitamins-and-minerals-older-adults
- https://ods.od.nih.gov/factsheets/list-VitaminsMinerals/

In addition to vitamins, our bodies require high amounts of particular minerals, including calcium, zinc, sodium, potassium, iron, phosphorus, magnesium, and iodine. Typically, 99% of the calcium in our body is used by our bones, and the remaining 1% is found in blood and other tissues. As we will explore in Facets, when the calcium levels in circulation decrease, parathyroid hormone (PTH) will be secreted and will signal the bones to release additional calcium into the bloodstream. Further, the hormone may activate Vitamin D to help improve the absorption of calcium in the intestines. Calcitonin, however, signals bone tissues to suppress the further release of calcium into the bloodstream. Calcium plays several important roles in the body, including maintaining bone health, blood clotting, and nervous system function.

Iodine is used by the body in the production of several hormones of the thyroid gland, including thyroxine and triiodothyronine, responsible for maintaining and regulating metabolism. Iron is most prominently used in the composition of hemoglobin, the protein found in red blood cells (erythrocytes) that binds to oxygen. Iron is the most essential component of the hemoglobin protein complex.

Sodium and Potassium are actively involved in controlling nerve impulses (particularly during the synapse, through the Sodium-Potassium pump in neurons). Sodium is additionally used in the maintenance of water and mineral balance in the body by regulating tonicity levels and protecting cells from gaining or losing excess water. Potassium is further used in regulating the -

fluid levels within our cells, whereas sodium is used to regulate the fluid levels outside of our cells.

Vitamins and minerals are yet another class of molecules that have been the caregivers of our physiology. With the necessary balance of biological macromolecules, vitamins, and minerals, an organism's physiology will be intact.

We will now explore one of the most significant molecules of our being, and the fascination behind the most important substance in biology. We will explore the molecule that governs our existence, our susceptibility to disease, and our reception of alternative stimuli. We have touched upon the structure and purpose of DNA; however, we will now explore its extreme relevance to our species and our future. We will explore the *genome*.

—

GENOME

PART TWO:

GENOME

"If we define "beauty" as having blue eyes (and only blue eyes), then we will, indeed, find a "gene for beauty." If we define "intelligence" as the performance on only one kind of test, then we will, indeed, find a "gene for intelligence." The genome is only a mirror for the breadth or narrowness of human imagination."

- Siddhartha Mukherjee

"We share half our genes with the banana."

- Robert May

Approximately 3.1 billion base pairs in length, the human genome has been a longstanding source of fascination for biologists. Further, a hallmark of prokaryotic and eukaryotic cells alike (from a bacterium to the cells of a plant or human) is the intricate, precise, and deliberate regulation of gene expression.

Surprisingly, until the 1940s, there was great debate between proteins and DNA as candidates for the genetic molecule of the cell. Even more surprisingly, the case for proteins seemed much stronger, due to heterogeneity and functional specificity, both hallmarks of hereditary molecules. In fact, the physical and chemical properties of nucleic acids seemed too consistent to account for the plethora of specific inherited traits exhibited by organisms. The essence of DNA's key involvement in heredity was first identified in studying viruses infecting a bacterium.

In the earlier half of the century, a British medical officer named Frederick Griffith was studying the bacterium Streptococcus Pneumonia, in search of any properties that could be targeted in developing a vaccine against infections caused by the microorganism. Testing two strains of the species (one pathogenic, the other harmless), he killed the pathogenic strain with heat, then added the remains of the cells to the living, nonpathogenic strain. Griffith was startled to find that, after some time, pathogenic cells started to appear in the previously nonpathogenic strain. Further, pathogenicity was inherited by all future offspring of the transformed microorganisms. Griffith was certain that some chemical component of the pathogenic strain caused this heritable alteration.

An American bacteriologist named Oswald Avery took on the challenge of identifying the transformational substance.

Focusing on three particular candidates (DNA, RNA, and protein), Avery extracted the cellular contents of the heat-killed pathogenic bacterium and treated each of his three samples with an agent that inactivated a certain type of molecule. When he tested each sample's ability to transform live nonpathogenic bacterium, he discovered that transformation only occurred when DNA remained active.

While Griffith's and Avery's work was instrumental to the identification of DNA as the primary genetic instructions of the cell, the discoveries were met with great skepticism, largely due to many biologists assuming genes in microorganisms would not be similar in composition or function to the genes of more complex multicellular organisms. However, years of discovery have allowed us to obtain a more clear picture of the structure of DNA, its interactions with its intracellular environment, and its role in the cell.

The DNA of eukaryotic cells is packaged with histone proteins in an elaborate aggregate called *chromatin* (composed of nucleosomes). The location of a gene's promoter (relative to the placement of the nucleosomes and the particular loci where the DNA is able to attach to the chromosome's scaffolding) will affect whether a certain gene is transcribed to RNA and subsequently translated into protein.

The strands of DNA in our chromosomes are wrapped around proteins known as *histones*. The modifi-

-cation of histone proteins can directly affect the regulation of gene transcription. Histone acetylation (the process of introducing an acetyl group to the protein) appears to open the chromatin structure and promote transcription. Adding a methyl group, however, will result in the condensation of chromatin and reduced transcription. Further, a different class of enzymes is able to methylate certain nitrogenous bases in the DNA strand itself (typically the pyrimidine *cytosine*). This form of DNA methylation occurs mostly on long stretches of inactive DNA, and less so on regions of actively transcribed DNA. Genes are more regularly methylated in cells where expression of that particular gene is not needed, and the these genes remain methylated through successive cell divisions in an individual.

To initiate the transcription of DNA into RNA, the *RNA polymerase* enzyme requires the guidance of transcription factors. While some of these factors are essential for the transcription of all protein-creating genes (known as *general transcription factors*), others are directed towards particular types of genes (known as *enhancers* and *specific transcription factors (STFs)*). The rate of expression of a particular gene can be significantly increased by the binding of STFs (either activators or repressors) to enhancers.

–

DNA, Histones, Nucleosomes, & Chromosomes

Strand of DNA

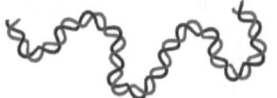

Nucleosome of 8 Histone Proteins

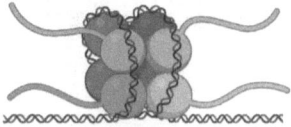

Chromosome of DNA

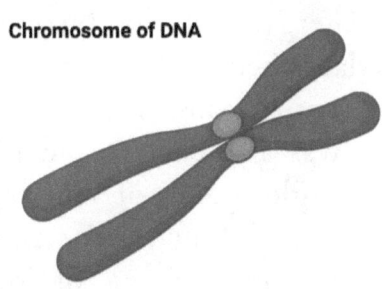

Deciphering the Genome

A founding goal of genetics has been to identify sequences of DNA that influence biological traits, especially ones related to the onset and progression of disease. In fact, for most of the ailments that humanity faces, our genetic diversity influences the susceptibility an individual bears to a particular disease. Until a few decades ago, efforts to correlate genes with disease progression focused on 'rare, monogenic and syndromic' diseases, driven by pedigrees and linkage analysis. This lengthy process resulted in over 1000 of the estimated 7,000 single-gene inherited diseases being characterized by 2001.

However, just a decade earlier, the United States Department of Energy and the National Institute of Health* formally launched a $3 billion (FY 1991) project to sequence the entire human genome. The Human Genome Project was launched to identify, map, and sequence every single gene of our species from a physical, molecular, and functional standpoint. One of the most seminal undertakings of our generation, sequencing the entire human genome challenged the greatest minds in biology for decades. Two technologies were central to the project's success: gene mapping and DNA sequencing. However ambitious the mission, the project proved successful. United States President Bill Clinton and Prime Minister A. Blair of the United Kingdom jointly announced in June of 2000 that the first-ever draft of the entire human genome had been -

---

* Throughout this book, the National Institutes of Health may be referred to as the NIH.

completed. Three years later, the entirety of the human genome was finalized, with the first printout still on exhibit at the Wellcome Collection in London.

Actually, the genome was broken into fragments, approximately 150,000 base pairs in length. Due to each individual having a unique 'genome', gene mapping involved sequencing a few additional individuals to get a more complete sequence from each chromosome. In fact, the mosaic nature of this modeled 'human genome' implies that it does not represent any one individual's genome, rather, it represents the idea that a majority of the human genome is consistent across the human species.

The sequencing of the human genome is a story of ingenuity, persistence, and global cooperation. It is one whose contributions to our species are limitless, and one whose completion represents one of the greatest strides in the biomedical field. In an article entitled *Genetic Code of Human Life Is Cracked by Scientists*, published in June of 2000, the front cover of the New York Times illuminated groundbreaking results of the project. The article documented: "The successful deciphering of this vast genetic archive attests to the extraordinary pace of biology's advance since 1953, when the structure of DNA was first discovered and presages an era of even brisker progress."

The Human Genome Project established that there are approximately 20,500 human genes. The NIH reports -

that the information could be thought of as "the basic set of inheritable instructions for the development and function of a human being". Francis Collins, then-Director of the NIH, shared, "it's a narrative of the journey of our species through time, an incredibly [meticulous] blueprint for building every human cell. And it's a transformative textbook of medicine, with insights that will give healthcare providers immense new powers to treat, prevent, and cure disease."

Discerning the Genome

How do our genes control who we are? How impact do mutations have on our physiology? In order to understand the functions of the gene, we must first step aside to review some basic terminology:

Genotype is defined as the genetic composition of an organism, while phenotype is defined as the set of observable characteristics an individual has. Think of genotype as the genes, or the DNA, and think of phenotype as the color of your eyes, or the darkness of your hair - the *observable* traits. An allele is one of two or more alternative forms of a gene or marker at a particular locus (point) on a chromosome

Chromosomes are long DNA molecules coiled in a double helix structure and wrapped up by histone proteins. And finally, genetic linkage is defined as the observation of two or more genes located on the same chromosome that are inherited together.

The processes involved in the transformation of genetic information into functional protein product is referred to as gene expression, and consists of two main steps: *transcription* and *translation.*

Transcription is when the DNA of a gene is transcribed into an RNA correlate. Particularly, this strand is known as messenger RNA (mRNA). The transcription of DNA is the work of multiple enzymes, including RNA polymerase, an enzyme that uses available nucleotide bases from the nucleus of the cell to form the mRNA transcript.

DNA, the double-stranded molecule whose construct determines our being, consists of a lengthy, repeated sequence of four nucleotides: *adenine, thymine, cytosine,* and *guanine.* As we explored earlier, RNA is similar to DNA in both its general structure and chemical properties. However, its structure comprises of only a single strand of bases, and uracil is the base used instead of thymine.

The next phase of gene expression is translation of the RNA transcript. Note that, between transcription and translation, mRNA splicing (or editing) occurs, where unnecessary regions of pre-mRNA are cut from the strand and only genes intended to be expressed remain. The edited mRNA strand makes its way to the ribosome of the cell, where it binds to transfer RNA (tRNA), a molecule responsible for "reading" the mRNA transcript and attaching amino acids accordingly.

In fact, mRNA is read three letters at a time, and each of these three-letter "codons" specifies a particular amino acid. For instance, the sequence of three bases - Guanine, Guanine, Uracil - correlates with an amino acid referred to as glycine.

Once a larger polypeptide has been built, the tRNA releases its amino acid and the remaining amino acids bind to one another, forming a long polypeptide chain. This peptide itself may be a protein, or it may bind with other polypeptides to form a larger protein.

Following synthesis, proteins are refined and packaged in the Golgi Apparatus of the cell. This process of gene expression, consisting of transcription and translation, follows the *Central Dogma* of biology, first proposed by Francis Crick in 1958. This central dogma, a kind of biological law, explains the flow of genetic information, from DNA to RNA, to make functional protein products, where RNA is the messenger that carries DNA's information to the ribosomes.

Proteins are the artisans of the operations of the cell. As we explored in Chaos, proteins are involved in a great variety of responsibilities within our bodies. Nearly every physiological process depends on the work of proteins.

—

In humans (as well as other organisms), particular traits are inherited, while others are environmentally influenced. For instance, eye color is an inherited trait. Organisms inherit genetic information from parents in the form of homologous chromosomes (a set of maternal and paternal chromosomes). If the DNA sequence at particular loci varies between individuals, the different forms of this sequence of genes are referred to as alleles.

—

If a mutation occurs within a gene, the resulting allele may affect the trait that the gene controls, and may alter the phenotype of the organism. However, most traits are more complex and controlled by multiple interacting genes within organisms. Many human diseases, such as cardiovascular disease and the various forms of cancer, are complex in that these diseases arise from the interaction between multiple alleles at varying genetic loci, with influences from the environment.

The purpose of the genome in humans is vast, yet incredibly necessary for the regulated survival of any organism, the carefully planned construct of its physiology, and the discernment of its future.

On a much larger scale, the proteins we produce serve crucial roles in the highly-specialized cells of our tissues and organs.

Yet we are still to understand the mechanisms behind the operations of these organs. It is for this very reason we must take this opportunity to swiftly examine our bodies' systems. We will now explore the aspects and processes of our body that facilitate our daily life. We will explore the intricacies of our biology - the facets of our physiology.

FACETS

PART THREE:

FACETS

OF OUR PHYSIOLOGY

"Life is not found in atoms or molecules as such, but in organization; not in symbiosis, but in synthesis..."

- E. Grant Conklin

We will now delve into the processes whose aggregate defines our physiological enterprise. These facets of our physiology steadily facilitate our daily functioning, and allow us to capitalize on nutrients and resources we find essential. These processes allow us to consume, hear, breathe, talk, smell, walk, talk, move, think, and respond. To start, let's explore a rather obscure community within our body - the *microbiome*.

Our Microbiome

The microbiome stands as a key interface between the human body and the environment, affecting our health in many different ways. There are actually as many microbes (bacterium, fungi, viruses) as there are 'human' cells in our bodies. This microbiome presents itself as both diverse and diffuse, establishing communities throughout the body, including the skin, gut, oral and nasal cavities, and other organs.

Our dynamic microbial community is largely formed in our primary years, yet differentiates over time in response to shifts in our diet, consumption of medications, and exposure to various other environmental influences.

To imagine the microbiome is to envision a bustling society of citizens frantically hurrying to work or making meetings on time. Think of the citizens of this society as thousands of species of microorganisms coexisting in our organs. In this case, "work" represents the numerous activities of the microbiota, whether it be breaking down toxic compounds or synthesizing vitamins and amino acids.

When we consume sweeter substances, while simpler sugars are consumed effortlessly by the small intestine, more complex sugars like starches travel to the large intestine, where hundreds of thousands of microorganis-

-ms help in breaking these compounds down with digestive enzymes.

The Human Intestinal Microbiome

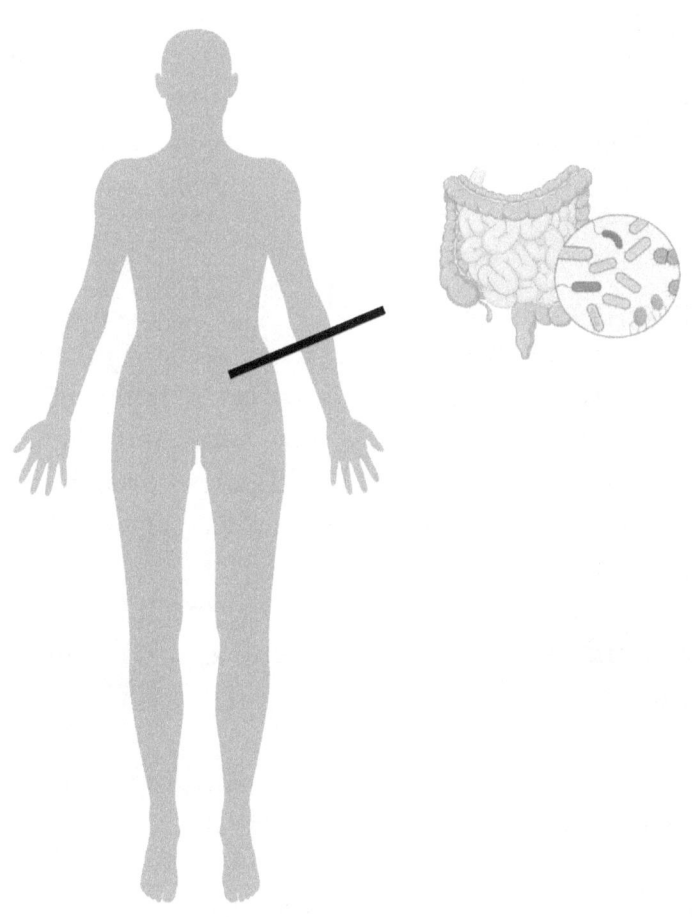

Digestion

The gastrointestinal tract (known as the digestive tract) consists of a series of hollow organs including the mouth, esophagus, stomach, small intestine, and large intestine. Being vertebrates, we are advantaged in that we have accessory glands, including the salivary glands, the liver, and the pancreas, as part of our digestive system.

Our digestive systems break the nutrients we consume into monomers small enough for our cells to use for energy and growth. Proteins are broken into amino acids, fats are broken into fatty acids and glycerol, and carbohydrates are broken into simpler sugars, like glucose.

During the cephalic phase of digestion, our gastric glands secrete molecules in response to the sight or smell of good. Once we ingest a substance, it is mechanically broken down and ground by our teeth, and chemically by digestive enzymes, including lipases (breaking fatty acids) and amylases (found in saliva, responsible for breaking carbohydrates like starch into glucose monomers). The process of chewing produces a bolus that is swallowed down the esophagus and into the stomach.

During the gastric phase, the bolus is mixed with gastric acid until it travels to the duodenum (the first part of the small intestine). The gastric acid released by the stomach consists of a class of activated, highly-acidic digestive -

The Digestive System

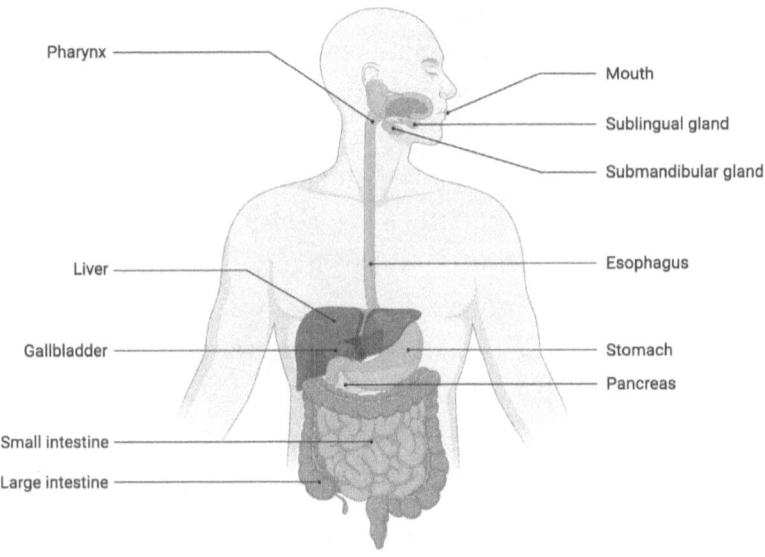

enzymes.

The final stage of digestion, the intestinal phase, begins in the duodenum. During this stage, partially-digested food, known as chyme, is mixed with enzymes produced by the pancreas. Chyme typically arrives at the small intestine one hour after a substance is ingested. In the small intestine, the finely-balanced pH and the addition of bile from the gallbladder transition the chyme into a state of alkalinity (or minimal acidity). At this stage, particles small enough in size and composition are absorbed by the intestinal wall and carried into the bloodstream. The large intestine, however, takes much longer to completely digest particles and remove unnecessary substances by defecation. As noted earlier, microbes in the large intestine assist in breaking down complex, nitrogenous substances. Ultimately, the digestive system converts the food we consume into its simplest forms, and transfers the nutrients into our blood supply.

Breathing

In order to make use of sugars we digest, we need to obtain another molecule: oxygen. As we explored in *Chaos*, our trillions of cells require oxygen every second in order to metabolize glucose, and obtaining the significant amount we require is not possible simply through digestion. Our respiratory system is designed to facilitate the gas exchange that provides us with sufficient oxygen for metabolism.

The reasons for breathing remained a complete mystery for centuries. A radically new understanding of breathing emerged in the late eighteenth century, however. In 1777, French chemist Antoine Lavoiser confirmed that oxygen represented roughly a fifth of air's volume, and that oxygen is necessary for the survival of animals. He also observed that breathing often released carbon dioxide. It became understood that breathing brought the oxygen needed for the combustion of food, and that this process would produce heat for the organism.

A more refined understanding of breathing emerged in nearly a century later, with the understanding of thermodynamics: respiration creates energy through the combustion of food, and this energy is used by the organism to produce heat and, more importantly, to power the physiology of organisms (including muscle contraction, activity of nerves, and synthesis of biological macromolecules).

The exchange of gasses in the lungs occurs in millions of small air sacs known as alveoli. This form of gas exchange occurs through ventilation and perfusion (the circulation of blood in the pulmonary capillaries). Our respiratory process involves cycles of inhaled and exhaled breaths, where inhalation brings air into the lungs. In the lungs, exchange of gasses occurs between the air in the alveoli and the blood in the pulmonary capillaries. Contraction of the diaphragm muscle results in varying pressures, and exhalation of carbon dioxide and other waste gases follows.

The oxygen we inhaled through our pulmonary vein to the heart, where it is circulated throughout the cells of the body.

Circulation

Many vertebrate organisms, including humans, have circulatory systems designed to deliver oxygen-containing blood to cells, tissues, and organs throughout the body. Our blood contains plasma (including hormones and growth factors, among many other molecules), erythrocytes (red blood cells containing hemoglobin), white blood cells (of our immune system), and platelets (thrombocytes, for blood clotting). Blood carries oxygen, nutrients, and hormones to tissues, and takes carbon dioxide and chemical waste away to the lungs for exhalation and kidneys for filtration. The bloodstream provides the stage for the activities of the immune system, and maintains homeostasis by stabilizing temperature and pH.

In fact, the composition of a single drop of blood is typically 250,000,000 red blood cells, 15,000,000 platelets, 400,000 immune cells, and 13,000,000,000,000 antibodies.

The essential nature of blood demands an entire system devoted to maintaining its circulation throughout the body. It for this reason that our body contains the organs of the cardiovascular system. The circulatory system includes the heart, blood vessels (arteries, veins, and -

capillaries), and is a closed system - blood is contained within the vascular network.

In preparation for tremendous criticism and disbelief, English physician William Harvey had accumulated a large amount of irrefutable experimental evidence in support of his stunning new discovery regarding the physiology of blood circulation.

Harvey had illustrated the processes of the heart, its chambers and valves, and concluded that blood moved from the right ventricle into the lungs through the pulmonary artery. Harvey's description of the heart's function and the aspects of blood circulation remain as a landmark medical textbook to this day.

The nutrients we carry travel through minuscule blood vessels and micro-circulate through organs and tissues. The heart pumps this blood to all parts of the body, where the left part pumps oxygenated blood returned from the lungs to the rest of the body while the right part pumps deoxygenated blood to the lungs through the pulmonary circulation. We know that heart is composed of two upper chambers that collect blood, and two chambers below that pump blood to the rest of the body. The valves of the heart let blood flow through the chambers of the heart and prevent the backward flow of blood.

The heart is the hardest-working muscle in the human body. At rest, an infant's heart may beat up to 130 to 150 times a minute, while an adult's heart often beats between 65 and 100 times a minute. In fact, the rate that the heart pumps blood gradually slows as you age.

There exists a diverse class of diseases originating from cardiovascular damage (damage to the heart and blood vessels). We will explore these diseases further in *Malady*.

Endocrinology - Our Hormones

Hormones are the chemical messengers that regulate and coordinate our many biological processes. Hormones are, in fact, the envoys of a much larger system. An entirely unique system whose presence is scattered throughout the body, often in the form of glands. Unlike the nearly-centralized organs of the cardiovascular system or the nervous system, you may find an organ of this system behind the neck, or beneath the brain. You may find one next to the kidney and another behind the stomach.

And anatomists have known about these glands for centuries. In 1856, French physiologist Charles Brown-Sequard conducted an experiment showing that removal of the adrenal glands resulted in the death of an animal, and arrived at the hypothesis that these glands contained substances that were indispensable to life. His work attracted great interest towards the secretions of the endocrine glands. The actual deciphering of the *hormone*, however, was made in 1902, when English physiologists William Bayliss and Earnest Starling observed that the duodenum stimulated the pancreas to secrete digestive enzymes regardless of connections between the two tissues, and coined the term "hormone", defining it as "a substance, produced in small quantities by an endocrine gland and circulated by the blood, that acts on another organ". A collaboration between Canadian physiologists Frederick Banting and Charles Best in 1922 yielded the purification of insulin, secreted by pancreatic islets.

While several earlier observations suggested that the pancreas was responsible for secreting an anti-diabetic substance, all attempts to isolate and purify that substance were unsuccessful, in fact, due to insulin being a protein and the pancreas happening to also synthesize digestive enzymes, such as trypsin, that serve in the breakdown of proteins.

To counteract the effects of the pancreatic enzymes, Banting ligated the excretory ducts of the pancreas, resulting in the death of cells involved in the synthesis of these digestive enzymes, all while avoiding any alteration of the secretory function of the pancreatic islets involved in insulin production. Unsurprisingly, Banting won the Nobel Prize in 1923 for his work on purification of insulin.* Around the same time, the first attempts were made at purifying the hormone involved in plant growth – auxin.

The endocrine system is a complex network of glands and organs, using hormones to control and coordinate our body's metabolism, energy levels, homeostasis, reproduction, growth and development, stress, and mood. While its organs are plentiful and present at multiple locations around the body, the most integral organ of our endocrine community is the hypothalamus, located at the base of the brain. The size of a walnut, the hypothalamus is rather atypical in that it is a part of both the nervous system and the endocrine system. In fact, the hypothalamus is the link between the two systems. The hypothalamus synthesizes and secretes neurohormones –

---

* We will further discuss the relevance of the breakthrough discovery and purification of insulin and the effects of insulin deficiency when we explore Diabetes in *Malady*.

that further stimulate or suppress the release of hormones in the pituitary gland. It is also directly involved in controlling water balance, internal temperature, sleep, appetite, and blood pressure. The pituitary gland is actually the intermediary between several endocrine glands. For instance, the hypothalamus may release a hormone to the pituitary, signaling it to release a hormone to the thyroid gland for secretion of, yet again, a third hormone at that location.

The *pineal gland* is located in the middle of the brain, and is responsible for the production of melatonin, a hormone whose presence in high concentrations signals to the body that it's time to sleep. The *thyroid gland* and *parathyroid gland* are located in front of the neck, and serve an important role in metabolism and in regulating the body's calcium balance.

The *thymus*, located in the upper part of the chest, produces white blood cells used by the immune system. The *pancreas*, situated behind the stomach, is involved in producing the key hormones *insulin* and *glucagon*, responsible for regulating levels of sugar in the blood and the subsequent absorption of sugars by cells in the body for metabolism.

Other endocrine glands include the ovaries, testes, and the adrenal gland (responsible for the release of corticosteroid hormones and epinephrine to maintain blood pressure and regulate metabolism).

While it may use *paracrine* (nearby-cell signaling), *autocrine* (self-signaling), and *neuroendocrine* signaling, the endocrine system primarily makes use of *endocrine signaling* - using the circulatory system to reach distant target organs.

Note that the hypothalamus is the most important organ of our endocrine system, involved in the coordination of several subsequent hormone release cascades. Its hormone products include *Growth Hormone Releasing Hormone (GHRH), Thyrotropin Releasing Hormone (TRH), Gonadotropin-Releasing Hormone (GNRH), Corticotropin and Releasing Hormone (CRH)*. Additionally, the hypothalamus releases a hormone known as *somatostatin*, responsible for inhibiting the activity of *Growth Hormone* and several other hormones. These molecules are the heralds for the production of hormones in the pituitary, including *Luteinizing Hormone (LH), Follicle-Stimulating Hormone (FSH), Growth Hormone/Somatotropin (GH), and Thyroid Stimulating Hormone (TSH)*. The many other hormones of the pituitary - oxytocin, prolactin, adrenocorticotrophic hormone (ACTH), and antidiuretic hormone (vasopressin) - each serve particular roles in the body. *Oxytocin* stimulates the contracting of the uterus and milk ducts, facilitating childbirth and oftentimes regarded as the *love hormone*. *Prolactin* initiates and maintains milk production in the breast during pregnancy and after birth, and TSH stimulates the synthesis and secretion of thyroid hormones. GH stimulates protein production affecting the growth and development of our body. *Vasopressin* -

regulates water retention in the kidneys, and is involved in the control of blood pressure.

The thyroid's signature hormone is thyroxine, involved in regulating digestion, heart and muscle function, brain development, metabolism (and the metabolic rate), and the maintenance of bones. The parathyroid gland releases Parathyroid Hormone (PTH), involved in regulating the calcium levels circulating in the bloodstream.

The adrenal glands release epinephrine (adrenaline), the famed hormone of excitation. Epinephrine increases oxygen intake, the flow of blood, and the rate of the heartbeat. Norepinephrine is released to further regulate blood pressure. Aldosterone is used to regulate salt and water balance, as well as blood pressure.

The adrenal glands additionally release cortisol, a steroid hormone that mediates an anti-inflammatory response and influences blood pressure. Cortisol is the stress hormone.

The thymus releases humoral factors that aid in the development of the lymphatic system (and immunity).

Interestingly, the kidney is regarded as an endocrine organ as well. Its cells produce *erythropoietin*, affecting the synthesis of erythrocytes (red blood cells). *Renin* works to control blood pressure by regulating aldosterone production from the adrenal glands, and *angiotensin* is responsible for the constriction of your blood vessels.

The Endocrine Glands

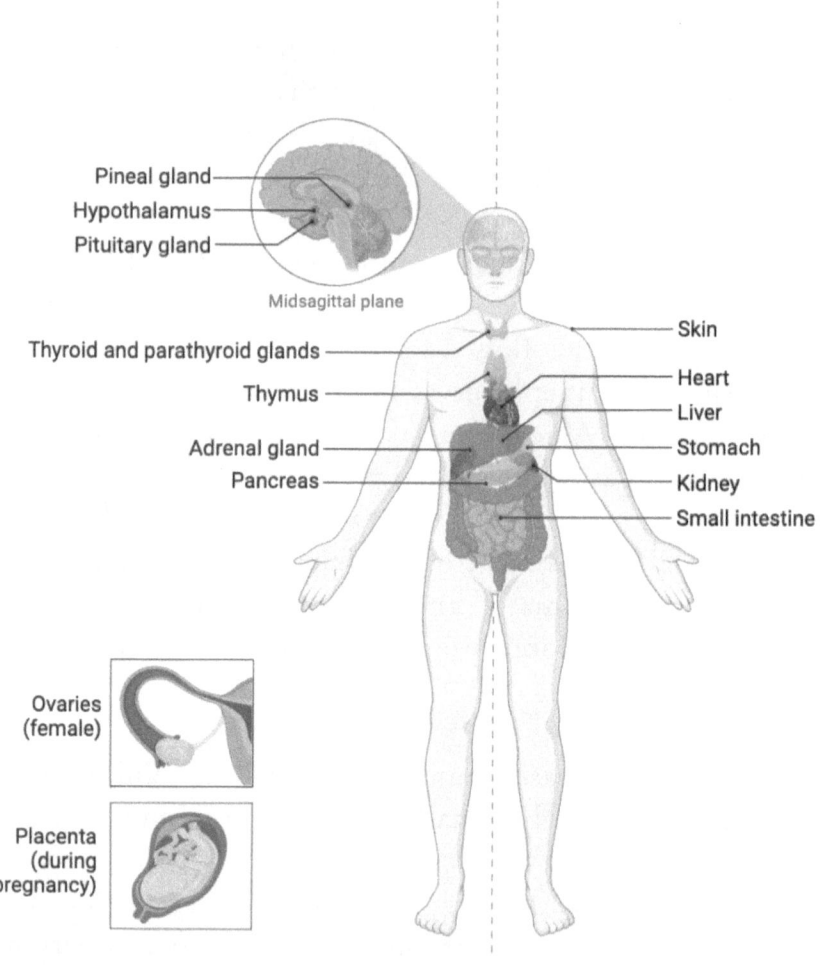

Needless to say, the endocrine system is a highly-intricate network that works to regulate and coordinate our body's physiology.

On the topic of endocrinology, let us explore a class of molecules intimately linked to the characterization of hormones.

Neurophysiology

In 1921, Italian physiologist Otto Loewi had isolated a frog heart placed in a particular fluid, and showed the the heart could be slowed through stimulation of the remaining nerve it was connected to (the vagal nerve). When he removed the heart and placed a second one, it was observed that the fluid in turn slowed the beating of the second heart, implying that a substance was released from the neuronal connection to the previous heart, and that substance had remained in the fluid and elicited similar effects on the second heart. While English pharmacologist Henry Dale later identified the substance as acetylcholine, Banting's experiment finally convinced scientists of the existence of a new class of molecules - *neurotransmitters.*

And it was the discovery of psychotropic substances nearly thirty years later that would convince the scientific community that the transmission of nervous signals at the level of the Central Nervous System (CNS) was chemical, similar to the signals of the Peripheral Nervous System (PNS).

The brain is a complex organ - one that controls our thoughts, memories, and emotions, as well as our touch, movement, vision, breathing, temperature, and, in fact, every facet of our physiology. Our brain is a conductor of the dynamic and flamboyant orchestra that is the human body. And yet, the brain itself is an orchestra of its own - an ensemble of neurons in synchrony, each with its own role in tuning (or modulating) the activities of the body.

Neurons stand as the cellular underpinning of our most prized organ - our brain holds an estimated 100 billion of these specialized cells. The brain - with its amalgam of neurons - comprises a part of the much larger *nervous system*. In vertebrates, the nervous system consists of two main components - the *central nervous system* (CNS) and the *peripheral nervous system* (PNS). Note that the *CNS* consists of the brain and the spinal cord, while the *PNS* consists of nerves that connect the *CNS* to every other region of the body.

The abilities of sensation and reaction actually originated billions of years ago in prokaryotes that could detect environmental alterations and respond in ways to enhance survival or reproductive success. Through evolution, improvements of simple recognition and response processes in multicellular organisms provided an advanced mechanism for communication between the cells of the body. Eventually, a complex nervous system developed in organisms.

In such vertebrate organisms, the brain and spinal cord are tightly coordinated. The brain provides the integrative power that underlies our complex behavior, and the spinal cord conveys information to and from the brain and generates patterns of locomotion, and independently generates reflexes (the body's default responses to particular stimuli). And in complex organisms, the axons of multiple neurons bundle together to form nerves - fibrous structures that channel and organize the flow of information along particular paths through the peripheral nervous system.

It's essential to note that the vertebrate brain is regionally specialized. The neural tube forms three anterior bulges as the human embryo develops. These bulges - the *forebrain, midbrain,* and *hindbrain* - together produce the adult brain. The developed brainstem arises from the midbrain, and the cerebellum mostly arises from the hindbrain. The forebrain develops into neuroendocrine tissues of the brain and the telencephalon, collectively called the *diencephalon.* The telencephalon later develops into the cerebrum, a region of the brain responsible for the control of skeletal muscle contraction and the center for learning, memory, emotion, and awareness. The cerebellum is responsible for coordinating movement and balance, and aids in learning and remembering motor skills.

Sensation & Movement

Our behavior is fundamentally based on the detection and processing of sensory information and the generation of motor responses. As we touched earlier, sensory receptors occupy many of our tissues throughout the body, and convert energy from stimuli to an alteration in membrane potential, regulating the output of action potentials in the central nervous system. Mechanoreceptors respond to stimuli including pressure, touch, stretch, motion, and sound. Chemoreceptors detect either total solute concentrations or specific molecules, and chemicals tasted or smelled. Electromagnetic receptors detect different amounts of radiation, while thermoreceptors detect surface temperatures of the body. Nociceptors respond to excess heat, pressure, or inflammatory substances and stimuli Photoreceptors in our eyes react to light stimuli

Most sensory receptors are in fact the modified dendritic endings of sensory neurons. Recall that all sensory stimuli is first sent to the thalamus for relay to the relevant region of the brain. The brain then activates motor responses through its musculoskeletal system.

The human musculoskeletal system is composed of bones, cartilage, muscles, tendons, ligaments, joints, and connective tissues, primarily serves to support the body's movement and in protecting vital organs, especially the heart, brain, lungs, and digestive organs. Skeletal tissue provides the primary storage system for calcium and -

phosphorus.

The skeletal system serves as a framework for the attachment of tissues and organs, and serves as a protective structure for vital organs. For instance, the brain is protected by the skull, and the heart and lungs are protected by the rib cage.

Further, our bones contain bone marrow, the primary location of new blood cell production. Where the yellow marrow is lipid-concentrated connective tissue (in fact, when carbohydrates are not available for energy production, the body makes use of the adipose tissue in yellow marrow), the red marrow produces around 2.6 million red blood cells (erythrocytes) per second in order to replace existing blood cells that have been destroyed by the liver. 2.6 Million blood cells per second is a staggering amount.

Renal Physiology

The kidneys serve various roles in the body, including maintaining acid-base balance (pH), fluid balance, sodium-potassium balance, clearance of toxins from the blood, absorption of glucose and amino acids, regulation of blood pressure (i.e. through renin), production of several hormones (i.e. erythropoietin), and the activation of Vitamin D. The *nephron* is the smallest functional unit of the kidney, and begins with a filtration component that filters the blood entering the kidney. The nephron then contains capillaries that reabsorb water and small -

molecules from the filtrate back into the blood, and the secretion of wastes from the blood into the filtrate.

The reabsorption of certain minerals, such as sodium, is stimulated by *aldosterone* hormones, and passive water reabsorption is stimulated through *antidiuretic* hormones. The kidney releases several hormones as well. *Erythropoietin* is released in the renal circulation in response to relatively hypoxic conditions (low oxygen environments at the tissue level), resulting in erythropoiesis (red blood cell production) in the red bone marrow. Calcitriol is the activated form of Vitamin D, and promotes the absorption of calcium in the intestines and the absorption of phosphate in the kidneys. For instance, when a significant rise in plasma osmolality (water-electrolyte balance in fluids) is detected by the hypothalamus in the brain, the posterior pituitary gland is directed to secrete *antidiuretic* hormone, resulting in the kidneys increasing water reabsorption.

Renin is an enzyme that regulates *angiotensin* and aldosterone levels. While the kidney is unable to directly sense blood, it is often depended on for the long-term regulation of blood pressure. When the renal blood flow (flow of blood to the kidneys) is reduced, juxtaglomerular cells in the kidneys convert *prorenin* into *renin*, and secrete it directly into circulation, where the conversion of angiotensinogen to angiotensin l occurs in the liver. Angiotensin l is next converted into angiotensin ll by the angiotensin-converting enzyme (ACE) often found on the surface of vascular endothelial-cells in the lungs. Throughout the body, angiotensin ll is a potent vasoconstrictor of arterioles – it is capable of constricting the passage of blood through the branches of the arteries, resulting in higher blood pressure.

The kidney is further responsible for maintaining a balance of glucose, oligopeptides (proteins and amino acids), urea, sodium, chloride, water, bicarbonate, protons, potassium, calcium, magnesium, phosphate, and carboxylate.

Interestingly, the kidneys are capable of producing glucose from lactate, glycerol, and glutamine, and are responsible for nearly half of the total gluconeogenesis (production of glucose) in fasting humans.

Homeostasis

In 1854, French physiologist Claude Bernard proposed the abstract concept of "milieu interieur", a kind of stability of the internal environment of an organism. Bernard's theories served as the underlying principle of what would later be termed *homeostasis*, one of the most important physiological needs of the body.

Bernard wrote:

> "The living body, though it has a need for the surrounding environment, is nevertheless relatively independent of it. This independence that the organism has of its external environment derives from the fact that in the living being, the tissues are in fact withdrawn from direct external influences and are protected by a veritable internal environment which is constituted, in particular, by the fluids circulating in the body.
>
> The constancy of the internal environment is the condition for free and independent life: the mechanism that makes it possible is that which assured the maintenance, within the internal environment, of all the conditions necessary for the life of the elements.

continued on next page

The constancy of the environment presupposes a perfection of the organism such that external [alterations] are at every instant compensated and brought into balance. In consequence, far from being indifferent to the external world, the higher animal is on the contrary in a close and wise relation with it, so that its equilibrium results from a continuous and delicate compensation established as if the most sensitive of balances."

Obtained from - Lectures on the Phenomena of Life Common to Animals and Plants.

By hypothesizing that complex organisms are able to maintain the internal environment (as well as the extracellular fluid), Bernard touched on the fact that homeostasis allowed for an internal environment to be regulated within a range of values compatible with life and to decrease the noise during the transfer of information and stimuli between physiological systems. Homeostatic factors include pH (acidity), internal temperatures, tonicity (water & mineral balance), blood pressure, mineral concentrations, and blood sugar level, and is maintained through receptors and feedback loops,

In 1932, a physiologist by the name of Joseph Barcroft suggested that higher brain function (and higher cognitive function) required the most stable internal environment, implying that homeostasis was not only a product of the brain - it served the brain.

The fundamental reason behind homeostasis is that the metabolic processes of organisms are only able to occur in particular physical and chemical microenvironments. The best-studied homeostatic mechanisms in humans comprise the regulators of the extracellular fluid, especially with regard to pH, temperature, osmolality, and mineral concentrations. In physiological conditions where homeostatic mechanisms are in excess or lacking, the terms *hyper-* and *hypo-* are used. For instance, *hypertension* is high blood pressure, and *hyperglycemia* is high blood glucose levels. Homeostatic balance is primarily controlled by the hypothalamus, and is often influenced by the circadian rhythm (a topic we will explore further in *Rhythms*). Our bodies are typically at the lowest temperatures during the night, and the highest temperatures in the afternoon. There are many other instances that involve our homeostatic balance.

Outside of the optimal pH range, proteins are denatured and digested, enzymes lose the ability to function, reactions are unable to occur, and the body is unable to sustain itself. The maintenance of homeostasis in the body may be the most crucial facet of our physiology.

—

While we will leave a discussion on two particularly large physiological subjects - our circadian rhythms (including our sleep-wake cycle) and our immunity - for the sections following, it is important to note that all of these processes are intertwined, with shared pathways, and operate in synergy.

RHYTHMS

PART FOUR:
RHYTHMS

"Sleep may be one of the most mysterious, yet crucial needs of our existence. Its innateness demands elucidification."

- P.M.

The circadian clock is our biological horologe. Its profound rhythm directs not only our sleep-wake cycle, but the aggregate of our natural tendencies and our most intricate physiology.

In some sense, our circadian rhythm sets the schedule for many of our most essential biological processes, and orchestrates effortless transitions within our physiological timetables. The circadian clock, interestingly, repeats every 24 hours, implying living systems have evolved and adapted to be in sync with the hours of day and night.

In fact, circadian clocks control the timing of a multitude of biological functions in organisms ranging from fruit flies to plants to humans. Circadian rhythmicity allows organisms to anticipate, prepare, and respond to precise, regular environmental changes. A riveting result is that organisms are able to better capitalize on environmental resources, such as food and light, conferring an evolutionary advantage.

An even more enigmatic question, I propose, is what drove circadian clocks to evolve in organisms? For years, scientists have thought that photosensitive proteins (proteins sensitive to light) and circadian rhythms may have shared origins. When considering that most DNA replication in multicellular organisms occurs at night due to higher levels of UV radiation exposure during the day, this hypothesis makes sense.

There are clear patterns of involvement with circadian rhythms in sleep, feeding (in mammals), brain wave activity, body temperature, cell regeneration, hormone production, and many other biological activities. The circadian system is additionally involved in photoperiodism, and in measuring and interpreting the length of day and night. Additionally, there is evidence of circadian rhythms predicting seasonal periods, availability of foods, an abundance of prey, predator activity, and weather.

However, the length of the photoperiod has been -

shown to be the most predictive environmental cue for the timing of physiological activity. In plants, instances of circadian rhythms are ubiquitous. Whether instructing a plant when to flower with the best likelihood of pollination or increasing photosynthetic activity during times of greater daylight, plants' circadian clocks regulate many integral aspects of their physiology.

In mammals, the primary circadian clock is located in a group of distinct cells known as the suprachiasmatic nucleus (SCN), grouped in the hypothalamus (region of the brain controlling homeostasis). Shockingly, a series of reports showed that damage to the SCN results in the complete disappearance of the sleep-wake cycle. It was established that photosensitive ganglion cells (neurons) located at the retina of the eye relay signals directly to the SCN, where the synchronization of the primary circadian clock occurs.

Further, independent circadian rhythms exist in many organs and cells besides the SCN, and are referred to as peripheral oscillators. In an article published in 2013, neuroscientist J. Takahashi stated that "almost every living cell in the body contains a circadian clock." Peripheral oscillators have been found in the esophagus, liver, lungs, spleen, thymus, pancreas, and adrenal glands, among several other organs.

Being such an essential component in regulating our physiology, scientists made it a priority to develop a fundamental understanding of circadian rhythms.

Sleep

The study of human biology is incomplete without delving into a rather whimsical phenomenon that pervades our existence - sleep.

Roughly one-third of our lives are spent sleeping. While we no longer wake with the chirps of birds and sleep with the crackling of crickets, our present-day sleep cycle is largely preset. Until fifty years ago, sleep was considered a passive activity, a state of being when the body and brain were dormant.

Matthew Walker, a famed professor of 'human sleep science' and author of *Why We Sleep*, shared in his book: "Inadequate sleep—even moderate reductions for just one week—disrupts blood sugar levels so profoundly that you would be classified as pre-diabetic."

Walker speaks of sleep in his book with great gravity, and warns of the profound consequences of a lack of it. Many aspects of our lifestyle we overlook often turn out to inflict damage so conspicuous in the long term that restoration of health may be difficult. This is the case not only for sleep, but for affairs so characteristic of our modern lives, including stress, inactivity, exposure to harmful lights and noise, and many more.

Each night, our bodies repeatedly cycle between two phases of sleep, known as Rapid-Eye Movement (REM) -

and non-Rapid Eye Movement (non-REM), 4-6 times. Non-REM sleep transitions us from wakefulness to restfulness. The three stages of this phase of the sleep cycle slow down heart rates, breathing, muscle movements, and brain activity. There is a slight drop in internal temperature. This is when the events of the day are processed and stored in our memory.

During the REM phase of the sleep cycle, brain activity increases, accompanied by increased breathing and a higher heart rate. The pupils of the eye twitch and move from one side to the other, the limbs are temporarily paralyzed, and dreaming begins.

These phases of sleep comprise complex underlying process that sustain our physiology and keep our bodies energized throughout the day.

Dreaming

We characterize dreaming as the succession of emotions, sensations, and ideas that occur in our mind (involuntarily) mostly during the REM phase of the sleep cycle. We humans spend approximately two hours dreaming each night, where each dream typically lasts between 5 to 20 minutes. While dreams may be fragmented and illogical, and were previously considered an epiphenomenon (a by-product of the neural processes we experience during sleep), scientists suggest dreams have an important purpose.

The evolutionary purpose of dreaming has been a largely unanswered question in medicine. Some scientists believe in the theory that dreams are meant to regulate emotion and deal with fears and worries, while others believe its purpose is to consolidate memory by replaying events from the day. Another theory suggests that dreams help solve (or forget) real-world situations we experience.

Each of these individual theories is understandable. The threat simulation hypothesis suggests dreaming serves as a simulation where we may rehearse threatening situations in preparation for an encounter. Additionally, there is very little evidence that individuals actually learn during dreams.

Caffeine & Sleep

A molecule with great notoriety, adenosine is a neurotransmitter that naturally accumulates in the brain during the day. When there is a high concentration of adenosine molecules bound to the receptors on the cells in our brain, a state of sleepiness is induced. Caffeine is a molecule often found in coffee whose chemical structure is nearly identical to adenosine. In fact, caffeine's mechanism of action is to inhibit the binding of adenosine to the receptor by binding itself instead. In an instance where caffeine has blocked enough adenosine from binding to available receptors in the brain, the state of restfulness is delayed and sleep is temporarily suppressed. It is for this reason that caffeine is the most used psychoactive stimulant in our society.

The levels of caffeine in circulation typically peak thirty minutes after ingestion. However, caffeine has a half-life of five to eight hours, indicating that five to eight hours after you have consumed caffeine 50% percent of that caffeine may still be active and circulating in the brain. Caffeine is eventually removed and metabolized by an enzyme known as cytochrome in the liver.

Caffeine is clearly a potent drug, and its effects on the brain and the body are relatively long-lasting.

—

Sleep Deprivation

Deprivation of regular sleep processes will fundamentally damage one's physiology. This isn't simply referring to the quantity of sleep; it's referring to the quality of your sleep as well. Signs of sleep deprivation include microsleeps (needing to suddenly sleep for a few seconds to minutes), reduced concentration, weaker memory and decision-making, slower thinking, and mood alterations.

Sleep deprivation in its acute sense raises the risk of unintended errors and life-threatening microsleeps. Chronic sleep deprivation, however, increases the risk of subsequent illnesses, including mental health disorders, immunodeficiency, and hormone imbalances.

—

Sleep, as we have touched upon, has a profound influence on the development and maintenance of the human immune system. But how does the immune system work? How do its constituents collectively carry out the defense of our being? As we explore the human body further, we must tour a network of cells who toil in harmony to achieve one fundamental purpose: defend the human body.

IMMUNITY

PART FIVE:

IMMUNITY

THE STEWARD OF OUR WELL-BEING

"Guardian of our health, gauge of our being."

- Anonymous

Where our internal systems power our daily functioning, we hold within us another particularly elegant network of cells. The often-overlooked guardian of our health, our immune system is a protective workhorse and literal bodyguard that employs use of complex, highly-intricate pathways to maintain our resistance to disease and our overall well-being.

Even at the level of the smallest organisms, a bacterium may have a special mechanism of defense against viruses or pathogens. Sponges, oceanic multicellular organisms containing pores and channels to allow for circulation of water, possess humoral immunity, a type of defense wi-

-dely considered as the first primitive immune response in animals. In fact, nearly all organisms possess some kind of immune system.

For many pathogens (whether it be a bacterium, fungus, or virus), the internal environment of an animal provides the ideal conditions for a habitat. Offering an enduring source of nutrients, a closed and protected setting, and a convenient system of circulation (bloodstream) for transport to new environments within the same organism, the human body is a wonderful host for a numerous variety of pathogenic agents. However, evolutionary adaptations have arisen that aim to protect animals against many pathogens.

Our innate immune system is the rapid, first response when we are exposed to a pathogenic agent. Our first line of defense, this class of organs includes the skin, the cornea of the eye, and the mucous membrane lining the respiratory, gastrointestinal, and genitourinary tracts. These organs help create a physical barrier against harmful germs, parasites, and cells. This part of our immune system is inherited, and is active from the time of birth. This system works to create a preconfigured response to broad groups of stimuli.

Our acquired immune system, with the help of our innate immune system, produces particular proteins, known as antibodies, to protect us from specific pathogens. Antibodies are developed by B lymphocytes. The antibodies that our B cells produce stay and circula-

-te in our bodies in the case that the pathogen is reintroduced into our bloodstream (getting the disease/infection once again). Immunizations train our immune system to produce antibodies after being exposed to non-harmful forms of a particular virus or pathogenic agent. In the event that we are actually exposed to the real form of the virus or agent, our bodies have already produced antibodies that are ready to target. This immunological memory leads to a more enhanced response to subsequent encounters with the pathogen, and is the basis for vaccinations.

We have T lymphocytes to directly attack foreign cells and produce cytokines, and B lymphocytes to produce highly antigen-specific antibodies. Our dendritic cells present antigens on the surface to other cells of the immune system, and our macrophages surround, engulf, and subsequently ingest foreign cells through a process known as phagocytosis. The natural killer (NK) cells in our bloodstream secrete cytolytic enzymes that break foreign cells apart. There are neutrophils and eosinophils and basophils. The immune environment is incredibly dynamic.

Additionally, the immune system is involved in regulating the physiology of our body. As we explored earlier, it interacts intimately with the endocrine and nervous systems, and serves a crucial role in embryogenesis, tissue repair, and regeneration.

Over a century ago, European zoologist Elie Metchnikoff discovered the critical role of phagocytosis and intracellular destruction in host defense, laying out the basis for innate immunity. After he studied simple organisms and identified specialized cells dedicated to the uptake of nutrients, he noticed these nutrients could be contained in particles, giving rise to the concept of phagocytosis. In 1883, he discovered that phagocytic cells were highly motile and were capable of migrating to different locations. Metchnikoff later suggested referring to these elements as *macrophages*, and became the principal agents of inflammatory phenomena that contribute to maintaining the integrity of the organism.

During a series of experiments on antiseptic activity of small molecules with Japanese researcher Shibasaburo Kitasato at the Institute for Infectious Diseases, he discovered that serum from infected organisms contained activity that was directed specifically towards the toxin from the bacterium. Around the same time, Emil Behring and Paul Ehrlich first identified antibodies as crucial counterparts to the toxic activities of the infectious microbe, responsible for neutralizing microbial toxins. This was the basis for acquired (or adaptive) immunity.

In 1904, Almroth Wright brought these mechanisms together by demonstrating a process he referred to as "opsonization" - the attachment of an antibody to a bacterium facilitating its phagocytosis. Many subsequent discoveries dechiphered the fundamental processes of the immune system.

All immune cells originate from the *bone marrow* and develop into specialized cells through a series of alterations occurring in different regions of the body. The common myeloid progenitor stem cell in the bone marrow is actually the antecedent to cells responsible for innate immunity - neutrophils, eosinophils, basophils, mast cells, dendritic cells, macrophages, and monocytes. The common lymphoid progenitor stem cell gives rise to cells responsible for adaptive immunity - B lymphocytes and T lymphocytes, as well as NK cells. T lymphocytes continue to grow and develop in the thymus.

These leukocytes are in constant circulation throughout the body, transported by the bloodstream, waiting for a foreign invasion. It's crucial to note that the lymphatic system, a network of vessels and tissues composed of an extracellular fluid known as lymph as well as several lymph nodes, is a conduit for travel and communication between tissues and the bloodstream. Immune cells sample the information brought in from circulation in the lymph nodes, and may activate, replicate, and leave the lymph node to circulate and target the pathogen if necessary. In patients, a swollen lymph node may indicate an active immune response.

While every individual antibody is unique, all are categorized into IgM, IgD, IgG, IgA, and IgE (where Ig represents *immunoglobulin*, the term for an antibody). CD8+ T lymphocytes (cytotoxic T lymphocytes) are critical for recognizing and eliminating virus-infected cells and cancerous cells. These cells contain granules wi-

-h cytotoxins that result in apoptosis. Due to its high potency, the release of these granules is highly regulated by the immune system to prevent autoimmunity.

And our B lymphocytes have two different roles: to present antigens to T lymphocytes and produce antibodies to neutralize infectious agents. These cells keep Major Histocompatibility Complex (MHC) molecules on the surface of the cell as carriers to present antigens to T lymphocytes. In response to antigen presentation, CD8+ T lymphocytes will recognize and destroy infected cells. Essentially, this form of *antigen presentation* precedes an immune attack.

Immune cells communicate with each other in several ways, including direct cell-to-cell contact or through secreted signaling molecules that bind to particular cell-surface receptors.

There exists a particular class of proteins central to the activities of the immune system - *cytokines*. These are the lesser-known heralds of our immunity. Certain cytokines, such as interferons and interleukins, are responsible for activating immune cell responses. Chemokines are responsible for attracting immune cells to a particular region of infection, and colony-stimulating factors are essential for immune cell development and differentiation. Tumor necrosis factors (TNFs) stimulate immune cell proliferation, activation, and subsequently, inflammation.

Our Immune Society
The Stewards of Our Well-Being

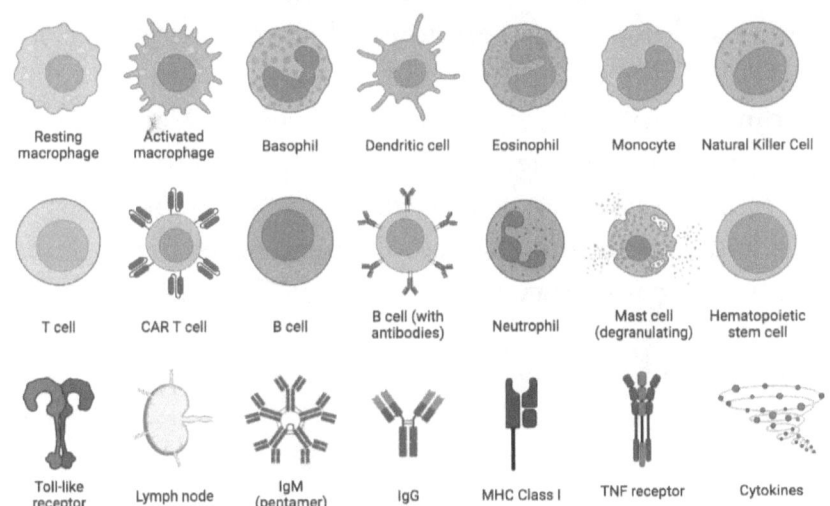

Our immune system is a diverse community of guardians whose aggregate stands to continuously sustain our health and functioning.

In the next part of this journey, we will study the very diseases that the human immune system is designed to face, as well as the ones to which the immune system is helpless. We will study the diseases from the most prevalent to the most rare. Diseases you've heard about and diseases likely didn't know exist. We will study cancer and neurodegeneration and hypertension. We will study diabetes and asthma and allergies. We will explore autoimmunity and respiratory syndromes. We will delve into genetic disorders. We will delve into the most treatable diseases, as well as the most incurable diseases. We will explore the essence of disease, and get to know our lifelong adversary.

We will study *malady*.

-

MALADY

PART SIX:

MALADY

"Let the [student] know that he will never find a book more interesting, more informative than the patient himself."

- Giorgio Baglivi

Of all issues humans encounter throughout life, few hover over our lives and, for some of us, impact every second of every day. However, nature has kept a particular class of adversaries extremely potent, a class that holds our very lives in its hands. This class presents its distinct, intricate forms through a familiar series of illnesses that attempt to weaken various aspects of our physiology. And while several of these illnesses arise from organisms other than ourselves (pathogens), many of these are a result of our own physiology malfunctioning on the basis of chance.

The human body is designed to deteriorate. To understand the most notorious of diseases we must first learn about the most understated of them all, one whose characterization as a "disease" may be astounding for many – *aging*.

Yes, aging may well be a disease.* In fact, aging is often *the* disease whose onset gives rise to a plethora of other diseases, including cancer, neurodegeneration, and cardiac disease. Over the past few years, several scientists have uncovered the underlying reasons why exactly we age. We now know the cellular and molecular alterations that underlie the abrasion of our organs.

The field of aging research has offered one crucial, surprising discovery about our cells. A process so subtle yet so fundamental to the diminishing effects of aging. A process that, if strategically manipulated or suppressed, may offer an end to aging, or at least a chance at significantly prolonging life:

Senescence

DNA, being a molecule requesting utmost delicacy, needs protection from the daily activities of the cell (being cell division and gene expression/silencing, in regards to DNA). At the very tip of a strand of DNA, there are thousands of extra base pairs with no true hereditary purpose, almost like a 'filler DNA'. The purpose of these unnecessary strands of DNA was largely unknown until the late twentieth century.

---

* According to several papers published by the National Institutes of Health (nih.gov), *aging* fits the medical definition of a disease.

Every time a cell divides, a small amount of DNA is lost from the ends of a chromosome. In fact, during every cell division, a chromosome will lose around 20 to 200 base pairs. Oxidative stress (the result of an imbalance between the accumulation of reactive oxygen species and the body's ability to detoxify these reactive products) accounts for the loss of another 50-100 base pairs per cell division. Telomeres are evolution's solution to crucial parts of our DNA previously disappearing with each subsequent division of the cell. Our telomeres are composed of hundreds to thousands of repeated six-letter sequences (TTAGGG* in humans). Telomeres are the protective caps on our chromosomes - base pairs with no genetic purpose, a kind of "filler DNA". When the telomere of a chromosome begins to shrink significantly, the chromosome reaches a "critical length" and is unable to be replicated. This triggers the cell to destroy itself through apoptosis, suggesting that the length and condition of the telomeres are indicators of the health of a cell.

One essential aspect of telomere biology to note is that the six-letter sequence (TTAGGG) is actually added by an enzyme known as telomerase. Alternatively known as telomere terminal transferase, telomerase facilitates the elongation of our chromosomes. It's the enzyme that increases the size of our telomeres. The catch is that telomerase is found in very low concentrations in -

---

* As we explored earlier, TTAGGG would represent the nucleotide sequence "Thymine-Thymine-Adenine-Guanine-Guanine-Guanine".

somatic cells (regular cells of the internal organs and tissues), suggesting a possible reason for why cells live only for a definite amount of time. Surprisingly, telomerase is found in high concentrations in germline (reproductive) cells, our stem cells, and tumor cells.

Cells that reach the critical length and are unable to replicate any further enter a state of inactivity known as "senescence".

Tightly packed into the nucleus of our cells, our DNA is constantly under a kind of chemical turbulence. The pristine carrier of our genetic information finds itself repeatedly encountering substances that could damage its structure or induce mutations. While mutations may be the result of the influence of several different environmental factors, most DNA damage is self-inflicted. Whether it be the chemical side effects of normal cellular metabolism or errors in DNA replication, the activities of the cells are oftentimes the reason for a mutation. While most forms of DNA damage are reversible (through an advanced repair process that detects for mutations), at times the DNA repair process may find itself impaired.

While proteins may last anywhere from a minute to an year, the average lifespan of an individual protein molecule will typically be 1-2 days. A key process -

involved in the recycling of proteins is autophagy (translating to "self-eating"), whose importance to the functioning of our cells was discovered with the work of Nobel Prize-winning Japanese scientist and researcher Yoshinori Ohsumi.

However, the body's impaired capacity for autophagy with age and its association with age-related diseases such as Parkinson's and Alzheimer's suggests that the process of protein recycling is a crucial factor in the aging process.

—

Proteins acquire incredibly complex and precise shapes through the process of folding. However, the exquisite intricacies of protein folding imply that even the smallest error in the process will result in a misfolded protein. Amyloid, a particularly detrimental type of misfolded protein, will often clump together with other amyloid proteins through binding exposed sections. Interestingly, a large group of amyloids bound together will form a structure known as an "amyloid plaque", and will strangle cells and tissues. Amyloids are found in the aggregates of Alzheimer's and Parkinson's as well.

The delayed, often error-prone recycling of proteins and the accumulation of amyloids leads to complications with proteins that are responsible for many of the issues we often experience as we age.

An interesting observation to note is that the increased presence of telomerase in cancer cells enables tumors to live and continue replicating indefinitely. If telomerase activity was suppressed, cancer cells would reach a "critical length" and would be unable to divide uncontrollably and indefinitely.

Cancer

Cancer is fundamentally a disease of uncontrolled cellular proliferation and growth. It's also a disease of resistance to apoptosis (cellular self-destruction) and of defects in the cell cycle. Cancer is a disease of trickery, evasion, and camouflage. Cancer is both the swine that exploits our biology for its personal gain and yet a remarkable instance of biological mishap.

Cancer is neither vulnerable to our natural defenses nor subject to the checkpoints and controls of the cell cycle. To give some context, the cell cycle facilitates the duplication of the components of the cell in preparation for division in the metaphase stage, where two genetically identical cells are created. The two key events of the cell cycle - DNA replication and the splitting of the replicated DNA - are a key factor in the uncontrolled proliferation of tumor cells.

---

[*] The following pages will cover the biology of cancer, and the mechanisms behind the disease. It goes without saying the cancer has been one of the most devastating diseases to go through, however, recent advances in modern oncology and cancer therapy have offered great prognosis for many cancer patients. We will explore these advances further in *Elixir*.

Healthy cells in the human body grow and divide in response to external signals, and cellular proliferation is controlled. However, when a cell develops a mutation, things change. Mutations can either happen spontaneously or through environmental influences, such as radiation, chemical carcinogens, or ultraviolet light. Most mutations are harmless, but some are powerful. In regards to cancer, the p53 gene is most commonly mutated.

This gene is responsible for tumor suppression (or preventing tumors from growing) by regulating cell division and signaling apoptotic proteins if necessary. Without the proteins for suppressing tumors being encoded, tumors can develop. In cancers, due to the loss of the p53 gene, cells gain deficiencies and continue to divide uncontrollably, not conforming to the cell cycle. However, p53 is not the only gene mutated in cancer. Similar to many genetic diseases, cancer is the result of many mutations across many different genes.

Benign tumors are harmless, but *malignant tumors* are exactly as the name suggests: *malignant*. Tumors of this form divide even more uncontrollably, evading the immune system and resisting apoptosis. Malignant tumors over-express *Vascular Epithelial Growth Factor* (VEGF) and thereby induce angiogenesis (the creation of new blood vessels) to supply the tumor with much-needed oxygen and nutrients.

And most notably, malignant tumors metastasize. Metastasis refers to the state when cells of a tumor have spread through the circulatory system to other sites of the body, resulting in the development of secondary malignant growths at a considerable distance from the primary site of origin.

Once metastasized, tumors are increasingly difficult to treat because of the spread to various parts of the body. If a tumor remains in one organ of the body and has not yet metastasized, it is less difficult to get rid of with the help of surgery or other chemotherapeutic agents. However, curing metastatic cancer is a very different story. Because it's difficult and impractical for a patient to have to undergo multiple surgical removals in different parts of the body, and certain times chemotherapeutic interventions are ineffective, several instances of metastatic cancer are incurable for particular patients. Even so, there are some interventions that, while don't cure cancer itself, delay tumor growth and reduce the symptoms. And cancer is not a *single* disease. It is instead a single term that comprises hundreds of different diseases, presenting itself in thousands of different forms. Whether a tumor originates in the *medulla oblongata* of the brain or the lymph nodes of the neck, each patient's cancer is unique. While most cancers are grouped by tissue or organ of origin, leading to classifications of tumor types, every patient's cancer requires a personalized response.

Tumors of the brain have been highly invasive. *Gliomas* originate in the brain or the spinal cord, and include *astrocytomas, glioblastomas, ependymomas, oligoastrocytomas,* and *oligodendrogliomas. Meningiomas* originate in the membrane surrounding the brain and spinal cord and are oftentimes noncancerous. *Medulloblastomas* originate beneath the brain and typically spread through the spinal fluid, and *craniopharyngiomas* originate near the brain's pituitary gland, affecting the pituitary's secretion of essential hormones. Cancers originating in the breast are known as *breast cancer,* and tumors of the lungs are known as *lung cancer.* And within each of these organ-based classifications exist subtypes. Cancers of the breast, lungs, skin, thyroid, and lymph nodes are among the most common among patients.

It is of crucial value to note that the prospects for cancer patients has drastically evolved in the past century. Once considered only a fatal disease, many patients of cancer now experience a regression of the tumor or an entire remission of the cancer itself. The advances that have made these prospects possible will be highlighted in Elixir. For instance, we previously discussed that cancers of the brain tend to be highly invasive. In this case, a remarkable class of targeted therapies and promising therapeutics have been developed that have improved patient outcomes.

---

* To learn more about advances in brain cancer, or other forms of cancer, I'd direct you to the National Institute of Health's pages on advances in cancer:

- https://www.cancer.gov/types/brain/research

Autoimmunity

The realization that our own systems of immunity might one day turn on us was a surprise to many scientists. While studying the immune system's role in the development of cancer as a medical student in the 1950s, Noel Rose discovered thyroid autoantibodies - antibodies that attack an organism's own tissues. Specifically, Rose found that a rabbit produced antibodies against its own tissue, after injecting an extract of the rabbit's protein back into its thyroid. The lymphocytes of the rabbit started to target the thyroid, and it was apparent that the body could, in fact, be attacked by its own immune cells.

Today, there are over 80 known autoimmune disorders, including type 1 diabetes, rheumatoid arthritis, celiac disease, and vasculitis. Autoimmunity is, essentially, our immune system targeting our own cells. The self-reactivity associated with these conditions often leads to tissue damage. While certain individuals are genetically susceptible to developing autoimmune diseases, genetically predisposed individuals don't always develop such diseases and individuals who don't carry any genetic susceptibility may. The main class of genes thought to be involved in autoimmune diseases are related to the synthesis and regulation immunoglobulins (antibodies), T-cell receptors, and major-histocompatibility complex (MHC) molecules, resulting in the of development of lymphocytes capable of self-reactivity. Certain infectious diseases may result in organism developing autoimmune diseases.

Neurodegeneration

In many ways, our memories devise our internal biographies, reminding us of who we are, what we've done, whose live we've touched, and who have touched our life. Needless to say, the loss of memory is equal to a loss of self, affecting every aspect of one's life. Worries about memory loss and declining thinking rank among the top fears as people age, in fact. What causes certain people to lose memory while others are able to retain it? While we understand that maintaining a healthy lifestyle may minimize our risk of developing many diseases and will keep our memory sharp, certain ensuing factors are oftentimes beyond our control.

Irreversible neuronal damage (referred to as neurodegenerative disorders) characterizes complex conditions that principally affect the neurons in the brain, leading to the progressive loss of neural tissues, including the death of neurons. Because our neurons are unable to self-regenerate after severe tissue damage, unlike the cells of our other tissues, and there is no known method to reversing the progressive degeneration of neurons, concomitant neurodegenerative diseases are considered incurable.

The most fatal neurodegenerative diseases, as observed in clinical studies over the last few decades, include Alzheimer's disease and Parkinson's disease, among various other cerebral failures.

The causes of neurodegeneration are vast, including abnormal protein dynamics (with defective protein degradation), oxidative stress and the formation of free radicals, impaired bioenergetics, and exposure to toxic chemicals. The most clinically relevant factors may, in fact, be inflammation and oxidative stress.

While much is already known regarding the genetic underpinnings of susceptibility to diseases such as Alzheimer's, there is still much to learn in order to translate this knowledge into therapies and treatments.

Diabetes

The food we consume is typically broken down into glucose and released into the bloodstream for the rest of the body to use. When the amount of sugar in our bloodstream increases, the pancreas is signaled to release insulin. Insulin is the hormone responsible for promoting the absorption of glucose from the bloodstream into cells of the body. Essentially, insulin is the key that lets glucose from the bloodstream into cells to be used for energy. Diabetes is a disease that results from a malfunctioning of this very process. In diabetic patients, the ability of the body to use insulin is compromised, one way or the other. It's crucial to note that there exists two forms of diabetes: Type I and Type II.

In individuals with Type I Diabetes, the body's ability to produce insulin is diminished. This is due to the autoimmune destruction of the beta cells in the pancreas. This kind of insulin deficiency is typically diagnosed by testing blood sugar or glycated hemoglobin.

Type I diabetes (T1D) is regarded as more severe and not yet reversible. The presence of particular antibodies (including anti-GAD) in the bloodstream have been shown to correlate with higher risk of developing T1D diabetes, and the condition typically develops in children. Type II (T2D), however, begins with insulin resistance. The body's ability to produce insulin isn't compromised; rather, the cells of the body are incapable of recognizing and responding to insulin's signals. T2D is many times reversible by implementing healthier lifestyle choices.

Symptoms of diabetes often include frequent urination (with increased ketones), increased thirst, increased appetite, excessive loss of weight, and vision impairments (or blurred vision). This vision impairment is often due to the buildup of glucose in the bloodstream, as observed in both forms of diabetes, that results in increased glucose absorption in the lens of the eyes. An individual with such symptoms must be diagnosed in time to prevent experiencing DKA (diabetic ketoacidosis), a life-threatening complication where the body excessively starts to metabolize fats and blood acids through ketones.

As a result of the purification of insulin (a life-saving breakthrough), significant advances have been made in the research for treatments and finding a cure. In recent years, diabetes has been increasingly manageable with the introduction of several diabetic devices, such as CGMs and precise insulin pumps, that have helped patients to regulate blood glucose levels, prevent DKA, and aid in the delivery of insulin to the bloodstream.*

---

* To learn more about advances in the research of diabetes, I'd encourage you to read the following articles from the American Diabetes Association and the National Institutes of Health:

- https://diabetes.org/about-us/research/research-impact/recent-advances
- https://www.niddk.nih.gov/health-information/diabetes/overview/managing-diabetes

Arthritis

Arthritis is classified as the swelling of one or more joints, presenting itself through symptoms including joint pain, stiffness, and decreased range of motion. Osteoarthritis (OA), the most common type of arthritis among patients, starts with the deterioration of cartilage (the flexible tissue lining the joints). When the space between the bones eventually narrows, individuals with OA undergo joint damage. Long considered a natural result of aging, the deterioration of cartilage in OA is oftentimes the result of additional factors, including injury, inactivity, and genetics.

Asthma

Asthma is an inflammatory disease that affects the bronchi of the lungs. The symptoms of asthma include wheezing, coughing, tightness of the chest, and difficulty breathing, and it's characterized by recurring symptoms, reversible airflow obstruction, and bronchospasms (sudden constriction of bronchiole walls in the lungs. Depending on the individual, symptoms may worsen at night or with activity.

Environmental factors that are considered to cause asthma in patients include exposure to air pollution, allergens, and certain medications. While there is no known cure for asthma, it is often treated by avoiding -

environmental triggers or suppressed with the use of inhaled drugs. Certain individuals with acute asthma will experience an asthma attack.

Asthma is the result of chronic inflammation of the respiratory tract (especially the bronchi), leading to increased contractability of the surrounding smooth muscle tissue and narrowing of the bronchioles. Interestingly, there is not one universal definition for asthma despite its high prevalence.

Genetic Disorders

Many of the diseases our species encounters are driven by genetic components. A genetic disorder is fundamentally any disease that is the result in whole or in part of an alteration in the DNA sequence of an individual. These disorders may be caused by a single mutation or by mutations in multiple genes along with environmental factors. Other disorders may be the result of damage to chromosomes or a decrease in chromosome count.

As scientists have uncovered the secrets of the human genome, it is getting increasingly clear that nearly all diseases have a genetic component. Several diseases are inherited from parent to offspring, while others are the result of acquired mutations that occur during an individual's lifespan.

Down Syndrome (delays in growth and intellectual disability), Cystic Fibrosis (damage to lungs and digestive tract), Achondroplasia (delay in cartilage bone growth and dwarfism), Sickle Cell Disease (atypically-shaped blood cells), Neurofibromatosis (disorder affecting the brain, spinal cord, and nerves), Hemophilia (the reduced ability of the blood to clot), many other syndromes, certain deficiencies, and cancers are all known to have genetic components.

Acute Diseases & Infections

Qualifying a disease as acute denotes that it is typically a recent onset and will not last very long. Certain viral infections, including that of the Influenza virus, and the common cold are considered acute diseases.

The bacterium *Staphylococcus aureus (S. aureus)* is present in our skin and the nose. However, getting the microbe any further into the body will result in severe health complications, including life-threatening skin, heart, and lung infections. Methicillin-resistant S. aureus (MRSA) is a particular strain that leads to complications due to its resistance to the antibiotics that are regularly used to treat such infections, making it increasingly difficult to eliminate from the body. Strains like these are known as "superbugs", spreading quickly in contained spaces and causing high rates of infection. Especially at risk are the patients at hospitals who often have weaker –

immune systems and and in whom a strain such as S. aureus can enter the body effortlessly due to cuts, wounds, and surgical procedures.

Similarly, *Escherichia coli (E. coli)*, a bacterium commonly found in the lower intestine, presents itself through more harmful strains – *Enterotoxigenic Escherichia coli (ETEC)* and *Enteropathogenic Escherichia coli (EPEC)*. It may be helpful here to remember that *entero* denotes the intestines. Pathogenic strains of E. coli may cause severe food poisoning, septic shock, meningitis, or urinary tract infections. The pathogenic traits in these strains are encoded by virulence genes.

These factors (or effectors) enable pathogenic microbes to achieve colonization of a region in the host organism, evasion and suppression of the host's immune system, and collection of nutrients from the host organism. In the case of ETEC, the strain produces two enterotoxins (toxins targeting the intestines), known as heat-labile (LT) and heat-stable (ST), that cause cGMP accumulation in the target cells and subsequent secretion of fluid and electrolytes into the intestinal lumen. EPEC uses an adhesin (adhesion protein) known as *intimin* to bind to host intestinal cells, resulting in a rearrangement of actin (a structural protein) in the cell and considerable deformation of the cells. The alteration to the intestinal cell ultrastructure is a key feature of the EPEC strain.

Cardiovascular Disease

Cardiovascular diseases are chronic conditions that affect the heart or blood vessels. Coronary artery disease occurs when the flow of oxygen-rich blood to the heart muscle is blocked or reduced, resulting in an increased strain on the heart, leading to cardiovascular damage.

When our diet largely consists of saturated fats, such as cholesterol, over unsaturated fats, our digestive system is sometimes incapable of breaking down the lipid molecules. When these large, saturated lipids enter the bloodstream, these molecules may clog the blood vessel and develop a plaque that impedes the flow of blood. This is a condition known as atherosclerosis.

The causes of many cardiovascular diseases are thought to be high blood pressure, high levels of cholesterol in the blood, mismanagement of blood sugar levels, inactivity, or genetic susceptibility.

Stroke

A stroke occurs when the blood flow to the brain is blocked, preventing the brain from receiving much-needed oxygen and nutrients from the bloodstream.

Within seconds, neurons start to die and neuronal tissue is damaged within minutes. There are two types of strok-

-es: ischemic (due to the lack of blood flow) and hemorrhagic (due to sudden onset of bleeding). Both presentations of stroke result in functional tissue damage in the brain, and signs and symptoms of stroke include a sudden inability to move, problems understanding or recognizing stimuli, and loss of vision to one side. Surprisingly, these symptoms occur soon after the stroke has occurred.

Similar to atherosclerosis, an ischemic stroke is typically the result of blockage of a blood vessel, while a hemorrhagic stroke is often the result of bleeding directly into the brain or the space between the membranes of the brain.

Respiratory Disease

Most chronic respiratory diseases are the result of either infection, pollution, or exposure to harmful substances.

The SARS-CoV-2 virus uses *angiotensin-converting enzyme* (ACE) receptors to attack cells of the lungs. A more general classification of diseases, pneumonia is an infection of the lungs caused by a microbial infection. There exists 30 types of Pneumonia, and hundreds of other infectious diseases affecting the lungs, such as *tuberculosis*.

—

Mechanisms of SARS-CoV-2

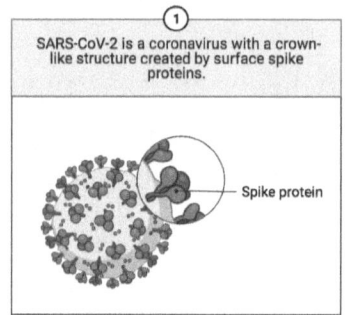
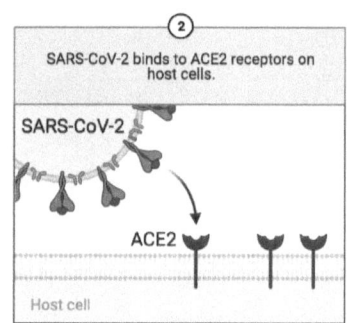
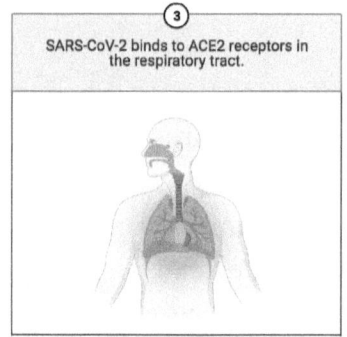
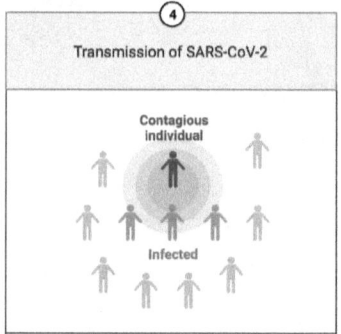

There are many other diseases our species encounters, far too many to delve into in this book. However, nearly every disease our species is faced with is being actively researched. It is quite reassuring to remind ourselves that scientists are actively working on treatments and doctors are committed to alleviating the symptoms of these patients every day.

Human disease has been a major motivation behind the study of science. Nearly every scientist or doctor hopes that his or her efforts will contribute to the overall well-being of society, and that the human species continues to thrive. In the next section of this journey, we will explore the concept of "cures", and we will study how human ingenuity has yielded great achievements in the ultimate practice of medicine. We will learn about how the body interacts with a substance (or drug), and how that substance interacts with the body. We explore the design and efficacy of therapeutics and vaccines. We will explore medicine in its most relevant form.

We will study *elixir*.

—

ELIXIR

PART SEVEN:

ELIXIR

"Wherever the art of medicine is
loved, there is a love of humanity."

- Hippocrates

Malady stands as an integral, darker part of our existence, but the essence of curative medicine is offering the light that illuminates our world once again.

From as far back as the earliest societies, forms of alternative medicine have been an integral component of prolonging life. These various forms of 'medical care' lacked biological plausibility, were oftentimes ineffective, and have not been rigorously tested, as compared to more modern medicines. While assessing the efficacy of certain forms of alternative medicine is a delicate subject because of its ties with many longstanding cultural and religious beliefs, it is widely regarded that most forms of prescientific medicine are not reliable in eliminating illness. However, the practice of medicine was clearly prioritized throughout the centuries.

Ayurveda

Ayurveda, a form of alternative medicine originating in the Indian subcontinent nearly 3,000 years earlier, is heavily practiced to this day. Ayurvedic therapies include herbal medicines, meditation, yoga, special diets, laxatives, and medical compounds, and preparations are typically based on complex herbal compounds.

In many ways, Ayurveda has inspired the current practice of medicine, or the "physician's art". Its famed eight components, include surgical techniques (*Salyatantra*), treatment of ailments affecting openings or body cavities (*Shalakyatantra*), toxins and antidotes found in animals, vegetables, and minerals (*Agadatantra*), rejuvenation (Rasayantantra), pediatrics and postnatal care (*Kaumara-bhrtya*), among others, and are interestingly analogous to our current approach to medical care.

Concepts of universal interconnectedness, the body's composition, and forces of life provide the basis for ayurvedic philosophy, and treatment often aims at eliminating impurities, alleviating symptoms, increasing resistance to disease, and increasing quality of life.

As the collective scientific wisdom of our society expanded over the years, so did our logic and reasoning behind designing newer medicines. Our society has shifted from the eras of herbal dilutants and bloodletting to more modern offerings of target-specific drugs or cellular therapies.

The practice of modern-day medicine has fundamentally shifted through a greater understanding of the biological mechanisms of disease. We now employ the use of logic, rigorous experimentation, and testing on model organisms more than ever before. These best practices have ensured maximal efficacy of what we put into our bodies to treat disease, and have eliminated many unintended consequences and side effects that have long been thought of as a necessary part of curative medicine.

Modern clinical practice entails physicians' personal assessments to diagnose, prognose, treat, and prevent disease using experience and clinical judgment. Modern-day branches of medicine are numerous, including basic sciences (anatomy, biochemistry, biostatistics, cytology, embryology, endocrinology, epidemiology, genetics, histology, immunology, microbiology, molecular biology, neuroscience, nutrition science, pharmacology, gynecology, and physiology) and medical specialties (surgery (i.e. cardiovascular, neurological), internal medicine (i.e. gastroenterology, oncology), medical diagnostics, anesthesiology, dermatology, emergency medicine, obstetrics, neurology, ophthalmology, pediatrics, and psychiatry).

Pharmacology

Modern-day medicine largely takes into consideration drug delivery. The principles of pharmacology govern the path a drug takes in our body, and are necessary to -

understand the series of interactions a drug goes through before having any physiological effect.

When a drug enters the human body orally, it first has to be absorbed into circulation, then distributed to various tissues throughout the body, metabolized (broken down), and eliminated or excreted in the urine or feces. When a drug is administered intravenously (through the veins), it doesn't need to undergo the digestion, absorption, and filtration processes of the gastrointestinal tract and the liver. Instead, because the drug is already in the bloodstream, it directly finds its way to the organ of interest in the body.

Once the drug enters the destination of activity, it will often bind to another molecule to either suppress or elicit an effect, or it will allosterically bind behind an enzyme or ligand receptor to prevent another molecule or enzyme from binding or activating any signals.

Other drugs act as ligands, binding to receptors, or specialized proteins located on the surface or inside a cell (intracellular receptors). The binding of the substance (as a ligand) to the receptor protein gives rise to a signal cascade, ultimately resulting in an alteration in the cell's function, such as boosting the production of a particular type of protein, slowing down DNA replication, or inhibiting the expression of a particular gene. In this case, when the signaling molecule (ligand) binds, it triggers a conformational change in the enzymatic domain to form high affinity binding sites for the second messengers.

Candidate compounds are selected as possible therapeutic agents for a particular disease of interest (discovery phase), and subsequently the compound is tested on cell cultures and animals, such as mice and/or rats, mainly to observe any tissue damage or side effects (preclinical phase). The clinical phase is when the compound is tested on healthy human volunteers, to make sure it's safe, and eventually on individuals suffering from the disease, to observe its efficacy against the disease.

This refined approach to drug design and delivery allows for more effective medicines and a more precise system for treatment. Modern-day pharmacology makes use of several model organisms that have remained true biological models and that scientists have relied on for hundreds of years.

Model Organisms in Research

While a model organism is any non-human species that is extensively studied to understand and follow particular biological phenomena, the genome of a select few organisms are closer than ever to that of humans. These model organisms are widely used in researching human disease at instances when human experimentation is unfeasible, unethical, or very complex. While the first model organism used in research is widely considered to be strains of *E. Coli*, researchers have been using the fruit fly for the study of genetics, mice for human diseases, and yeast for molecular and cellular biology for many years. In fact, discoveries made in these model organisms have yielded some of the largest breakthroughs in the medical field.

The genome of all major model organisms have been sequenced, and several databases provide researchers with the entire DNA/RNA sequences and protein transcripts. In other instances, researchers utilize cell culture, where individual cells extracted from an organism are grown under controlled conditions in vivo, in the lab.

Model organisms have brought some of the greatest insights into biology and medicine. For instance, countless discoveries made in mice, fruit flies, and yeast have earned scientists the Nobel Prize.

Notable Model Organisms in Research

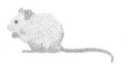 ***Mus Musculus* (Mouse)**

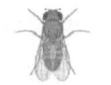 ***Drosophila Melanogaster* (Fruit Fly)**

  Saccharomyces Cerevisiae (Yeast)

Surgery

For centuries, a famed medical operation has been the surgical procedure.

Presently, surgery is used for many purposes, whether it be taking a biopsy of a lump or growth, further exploring the condition of an organ before making a diagnosis, removing or repairing damaged tissues and organs, removing objects that cause obstruction or impede blood flow, reposition organs and body structures, redirect blood vessels, implant medical devices, or transplanting an entirely new tissue or organ.

Minimally invasive surgeries do not require large incisions, allowing patients to recuperate faster with minimal pain. These include laparoscopy, endoscopy, arthroscopy, bronchoscopy, thoracoscopy, hysteroscopy, and laryngoscopy, among others.

Open surgeries, however, involve cutting the skin and subsequent tissues until an entire organ or tissue of interest is visible and operable.

While an intervention regularly practiced for centuries, the surgical procedure has been a very risky endeavor, both for the patient and for the surgeon. More obviously, the process of cutting into a patient's body is extremely pain-inducing, and the trauma of the procedure itself may injure an individual.

Anesthetics

Because of the invasiveness and extreme pain often occurring as a by-product of a surgical procedure, surgery has often been a treatment of last resort for patients until the 19th century. Two great advances, however, have made the operation of surgery almost painless, allowing patients to often survive the procedure.

In addition to the development and application of modern antiseptic techniques in surgery (preventing the risk of infection or sepsis), the introduction of anesthetic agents transformed the practice of surgery.

The first attempts at general anesthesia were, of course, herbal. Since then, however, the fields of pharmacology and chemistry have introduced more refined agents of anesthesia.

Many of us can relate to the experience of drifting into a state of unconsciousness before a surgery or medical operation following inhalation or injection of an anesthetic. But what happens while we are unconscious? How does anesthesia work? And how are we able to regain consciousness?

Administering anesthesia is a highly risky endeavor. Too much is dangerous, but too little and a patient can be left aware of the procedure and unable to communicate that awareness.

Anesthesiologists have to perfect just the right dose; otherwise, the drug can have detrimental consequences on the patient. Anesthetics are drugs used to induce a temporary loss of sensation or awareness, and come in two categories: general anesthetics (facilitating reversible loss of consciousness) and local anesthetics (facilitating loss of sensation for a limited region of the body without necessarily affecting consciousness). Some examples of anesthetics include fentanyl, propofol, ketamine, and cocaine, among over 110 others. Many times, clinicians will choose a combination of drugs to achieve the degree of anesthesia characteristics appropriate for the type of procedure, including hypnotics, dissociatives, sedatives, adjuncts, narcotics, analgesics, and neuromuscular-blocking drugs, in addition to general or local anesthetics. The three aspects of administering anesthesia that require the most attention are 1) the health of the patient, 2) the complexity (and stress) of the procedure itself, and 3) the anesthetic technique.

When inducing anesthesia, perioperative risks may be fatal, emphasizing the importance of a well-trained anesthesiologist during a surgery. Patients under anesthesia must undergo continuous physiological monitoring, including electrocardiography (ECG), metrics of heart rate, blood pressure, blood oxygen saturation, and body temperature, ensuring the safety and health of the patient during the procedure.

Anesthetic medications are usually delivered either intravenously or through inhalation by mask. Once sedated, the anesthesiologist may insert a tube into the patient's mouth and down the windpipe, ensuring that the patient receives enough oxygen and the lungs are protected from blood and other body fluids.

Despite the knowledge regarding how anesthetics work, the scientific community still regards consciousness as a mystery. Decades of developments have transformed surgery from a horrific ordeal into a "gentle slumber", but how exactly do anesthetics affect our consciousness and sensation?

Anesthetics work by interrupting nerve signals in the patient's brain and body to prevent the brain from processing pain and remembering what happened during the procedure. The drugs target proteins in the membranes around neurons. Scientists understand that inhaled anesthetics and intravenous anesthetics target different sets of proteins, but ultimately both block nerve transmission to pain centers in the central nervous system by binding to and inhibiting the function of sodium-ion channels. This inhibition of nerve transmission produces a loss of sensation and awareness.

Even with this knowledge, many aspects of anesthesia and consciousness remain unclear. For instance, it is still unknown how exactly nerve blocks result in loss of consciousness.

Antibiotics & Antivirals

In 1928, a striking discovery was made that led to the widespread use of antibiotics. While antibiosis was first observed in 1877 by Louis Pasteur and Robert Koch, whereby an airborne bacillus was able to inhibit the growth of Bacillus anthracis, Alexander Fleming's work effectively heralded the emergence of the antibiotic age.

Upon returning from a holiday, Fleming began sorting through Petri dishes that contained colonies of *Staphylococcus*, a bacterium known for causing sore throats. One particular petri dish contained a growing region of mold, amidst the visibly-dotted colonies comprising the remaining area of the dish. There was a zone immediately around the mold that appeared clear of any microbial growth. It appeared that the mold had secreted a substance that had inhibited the growth of any colonies in that zone.

Before this mold was later identified as a rare strain of Penicillium notatum, Fleming had observed that the mold was capable of inhibiting the growth of several other microorganisms, including Streptococcus and Meningococcus.

Antimicrobial resistance (referred to as antibiotic resistance) occurs when microbes no longer respond to antibiotics after evolving mechanisms that protect them from the effects of antimicrobials, making it increasingly difficult to treat diseases without antibiotics.

A group of researchers (including Howard Florey, Ernst Chain, and colleagues) are in fact credited with transforming penicillin from a laboratory curiosity into a life-saving antibiotic. This group worked on the purification of penicillin for medical use. Antibiotics have since evolved into the most effective type of antimicrobial agent for fighting microbial infections.

On a similar note, antivirals are a class of medical drugs used for treating infections resulting from viruses and focus on inhibiting a virus' development rather than destroying the pathogen. Currently, antivirals have been developed to treat infections of the Human Immunodeficiency Virus, Herpes virus, Influenza virus, and Hepatitis B virus. While researchers are actively working to extend the range of antivirals to other families of pathogens, designing safe and effective antivirals is extremely difficult due to any virus' ability to use the host's cells to replicate as well as the variety of viruses, making it difficult to find targets without harming the host organism's cells.

Stem Cell Therapy

Recall that a stem cell is a cell with the unique ability to develop one of several specialized cell types. Stem cells provide both new cells for the growing body as well as replacement of specialized cells that are damaged. Two defining characteristics of these cells include the ability to divide indefinitely and the ability to specialize upon cell division.

In addition to helping us understand the biology of living systems, stem cells may be used therapeutically. Stem cell therapy aims to replace damaged tissue that our body is incapable of replacing, and comprises the generation of new cells that may then be transplanted into the body to replace damaged tissues. Currently, blood stem cells are offered to provide a healthy source of blood tissue for patients with blood-related health conditions, such as thalassemia, as well as cancer patients who may be anemic. Bone marrow transplants (hematopoietic stem cell transplants), widely regarded as the most successful stem cell therapy as of now, have been offered for more than 40 years. Transplanted bone marrow may be used to replace damaged bone marrow (conditions such as aplastic anemia), regenerate a new immune system that will fight existing or residual tumors, restore the function of bone marrow after high doses of chemotherapy are administered, or to replace it with genetically healthy bone marrow to prevent further damage from a genetic disease (such as adrenoleukodystrophy).

Genetic Engineering

By the 1970s, a group of scientists (including W. Arber and H. Smith) had discovered that the restriction observed in bacteriophages was the result of an enzymatic cleavage of DNA. These restriction enzymes were defense mechanisms used by many microorganisms against viruses, effectively cutting foreign DNA while host DNA was protected by modification enzymes. Further, the ability of restriction enzymes to cut DNA at precise locations posed great potential for manipulation.

This discovery had entirely altered the landscape of molecular biology, and had broadened scientists' expectations of the capabilities of an entirely new discipline: genetic engineering.

With the discovery of restriction enzymes, along with that of vectors (small DNA molecules enabling genes to be cloned), techniques for sequencing and directing the induction of mutations in DNA had been developed.
And in 1974, a scientist by the name of Rudolf Jaenisch introduced foreign DNA into the embryos of a mouse, and created the first genetically modified animal.

Genetic engineering (or gene editing) refers to the ingenious method of altering the genetic instruction of an organism by either removing or introducing DNA, and has the potential to fix severe genetic disorders by effectively replacing the defective (or mutated) gene with a functional alternative.

In 1976, the world's first genetic engineering company - *Genentech* - was founded. Within a year, the company had produced the human *somatostatin* protein in cells of E. coli. Further, Genentech announced success in producing human insulin through genetically-engineered microorganisms in culture. This modified form of insulin - *humulin* - was licensed for use by humans in 1982.

The particular mechanisms behind genetic engineering are not incredibly difficult to understand. Typically, a small circular strand of DNA (referred to as a plasmid) is extracted from a bacterium or yeast cell. A particular region of the DNA strand is cut with restriction enzymes, a kind of "molecular scissors". A functional gene of interest (such as the gene for insulin in humans) is introduced to the plasmid, resulting in a *genetic modification*. Following the central dogma of biology (DNA makes RNA, and RNA makes protein), this genetically-modified strand of DNA is reproduced in daughter cells of the microorganism, and the gene is expressed, resulting in the production of a particular protein. In the case of insulin, the mixture of cells are filtered to release the insulin protein, and subsequently purified and distributed to patients with diabetes.

The Genetic Engineering Process

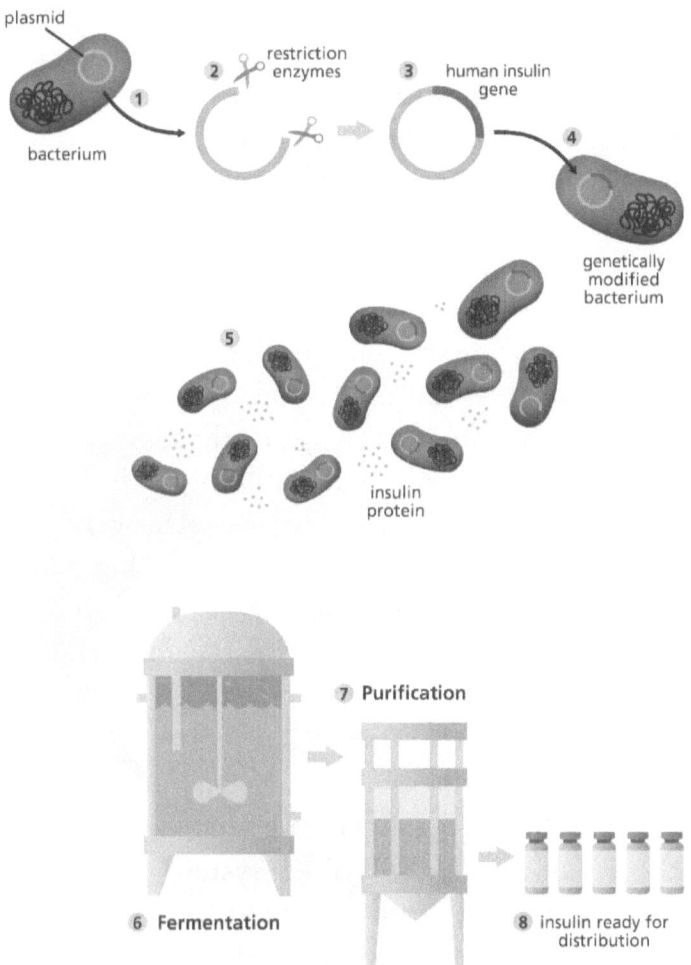

Image Credit: Genome Research Limited

The applications of genetic engineering are numerous. In addition to the production of particular proteins and hormones, genetic engineering has been applied to plants to improve the resilience, nutritional value, and growth rate of several crops. Sheep have been genetically engineered to produce a protein through milk that may be used to treat cystic fibrosis, and the genomes of smaller organisms have been altered to mutate and follow the expression patterns of genes associated with Alzheimer's disease.

Several other techniques, more relevant to the study of the biology of a disease rather than its treatment, have offered innovative methods of gene editing. The inactivation of an organism's genes through homologous recombination (referred to as "knocking out a gene"), and the use of RNA interference to selectively inhibit a gene's expression (referred to as "knocking down a gene") together have significantly contributed to our understanding of the functions of particular genes.

CRISPR

One of the most significant advances in medicine has been the use of the CRISPR-Cas9 system in gene editing. Awarded the Nobel Prize in 2020, American scientist Jennifer Doudna and French microbiologist Emmanuelle Charpentier published findings in 2012 that the CRISPR-Cas9 system could be genetically programmed with RNA to edit genomic DNA.

Mechanisms Behind CRISPR-Cas9 System

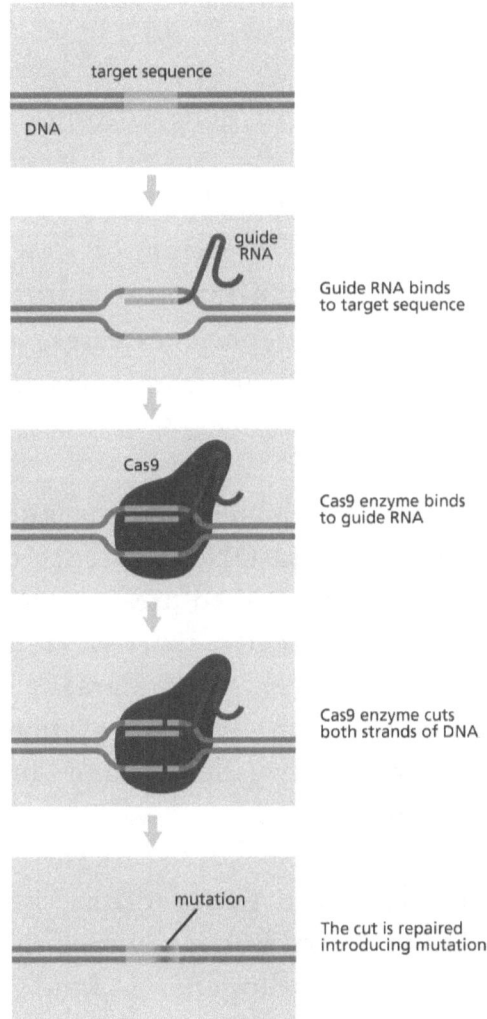

Image Credit: Genome Research Limited

By delivering the Cas9 nuclease with a synthetic guide RNA molecule, any cell's genome may be cut at a particular location of interest, allowing existing genes to be removed and new ones to be added *in vivo*.

This particular method of gene editing allows for an organism's genome to be edited *in vivo* (in the organism itself) with extremely high precision, and its applications include the creation of new medicines, genetically modified organisms, agricultural products, treatment of inherited genetic diseases, and possible treatment of diseases arising from somatic mutations, including cancer.

Another kind of genetic scissors, the nuclease opens both strands of a targeted DNA sequence to introduce the modification. Compared to previous forms of gene editing in eukaryotic cells that were often times inefficient or impractical to implement on a large scale, researchers using the CRISPR system are able to efficiently and precisely silence and induce point mutations at particular loci.

Certain microbes have gene editing systems using CRISPR, and like restriction enzymes, this system is used to respond to pathogens, a kind of immune system. The modern CRISPR-Cas9 system is derived from this microbial defense mechanism.

Several proposed applications of the CRISPR system in humans involved editing the genomes of germline reproductive) cells. Because any alterations made in these cells will be inherited by an organism's offspring, this application of the CRISPR system bears great ethical concern. However, it may be an extremely effective way of eliminating future generations from inheriting a family's known genetic disorder.

While it's likely going to be a long time before the CRISPR system will be used routinely in humans, great strides have been made in its discovery and current applications.

Aging Research

Developing a cure for aging will likely require a significant reprogramming of our biology. Scientists have observed that mutations in single genes may entirely alter the lifespan of mice and other model organisms in the lab. There must be a way to observe similar effects in humans.

Geneticists have found that certain genes are overexpressed in individuals who live to be 100 years in age or elder. Two genes in particular - *APOE* and *FOXO3* - offered striking correlations. The *APOE* gene encodes for a protein responsible for transporting cholesterol throughout the body, and the *FOXO3* gene is transcribed and subsequently translated into a protein responsible for triggering apoptotic pathways in cells.

Another method scientists are considering and actively researching is turning back the epigenetic clock. An interesting fact to note is that, regardless of the age of a baby's parents, he or she is born young, at the age of zero. Babies inherit the DNA from parents, and yet do not inherit either parent's chronological age. Nature, in fact, has made the germline immortal. The cells of the germline, involved in reproduction, will never age because these cells are the sole determinants of the continuity of a species. Several researchers have found that induced pluripotent stem cells (iPSCs) appear to rejuvenate cells in ways that mimic how nature offers babies youth.

Where the epigenetic clock is clearly an accurate predictor of biological age based on epigenetic marks on your DNA, testing the epigenetic clock of iPSCs indicated that these cells were epigenetically zero years of age, similar to embryonic cells.

While the journey from lab research to clinical medicine is often extremely difficult and lengthy (many brilliant ideas prove to be a puzzle to put into practice), there are several reasons to stay optimistic. Researchers have found several different ways to extend the healthy lifespan of mice, including dietary restrictions, telomerase, and senolytics.

Aging is not inevitable; it is instead highly reversible. While a simple "cure" - a one-time treatment that wo-

-uld completely prevent the body from aging - may not be feasible given our current understanding of aging biology and the need for an entire reprogramming of human biology, increasing life expectancy, however, through suppressing the intricacies of the aging process piece by piece is certainly likely. While the diabetes drug metformin is a significant contender to delay the aging process, future clinical experimentation will offer a clearer picture of its efficacy.

Currently, humans are able to take various steps that may increase life expectancy. It is essential to limit your exposure to toxic chemicals, gasses, and products; these substances may induce mutations in your DNA and chronic inflammation. Eating more fruits and vegetables has been shown to increase the diversity of your microbiome, and obtaining your protein from plant sources may serve similar effects as dietary restriction. An experiment in 1987 by the National Institute on Aging showed that monkeys fed a regular diet lived to be 21 years without disease, while the group of monkeys who had undergone diet restrictions had an extra five years or more free of disease. Translating these results into human years, that's an extra ten years or more free from age-related illnesses. Intermittent fasting or skipping a meal a day after the age of 50 has shown a great correlation with increased lifespan in patients. Further, dietary restrictions improve markers of health, including blood pressure, cholesterol levels, and inflammation levels. While we shouldn't deprive ourselves of essential nutrients and minerals, intermittent fasting may offer benefits in the long run.

Another key finding in nutrition has been that excess fat deposits (adipose tissues) are not healthy, increasing your susceptibility to cardiovascular disease. Reducing your sugar consumption will reduce the quantity of glycated protein. Getting enough hours of sleep each day, as we explored in Rhythms, will create a stable sleep rhythm that may factor into a more robust immune system. Monitoring your heart rate and blood pressure will keep you aware of any potential cardiovascular complications.

And unless you have a particular vitamin deficiency requiring the ingestion of supplements, clinical evidence doesn't yet support the use of vitamins for healthy individuals. In patients of a large clinical study of 300,000 healthy individuals, researchers found vitamin supplements had no effect on the risk of illness, and in the case of beta-carotene (what the body converts into Vitamin A) and Vitamin E, individuals had a slightly increased risk of developing illnesses.

—

Chemotherapy & Targeted Therapy

Of course, one of the most puzzling and consuming diseases humanity has faced may well be cancer. The medical field has attempted to "cure" the human body of cancer for centuries. From the earliest attempts at surgically removing the tumor to the modern attempts of targeting cancer cells with chemotherapy, the search for a "cure" for cancer, as if it were a single disease capable of being "cured", has been a focus for scientists and doctors for centuries.

—

Siddhartha Mukherjee, a well-known oncologist, scientist, and writer, once wrote: "Cancer chemotherapy, consumed by its fiery obsession to obliterate the cancer cell, found its roots in the obverse logic: every poison might be a drug in disguise". In many ways, this well characterizes the first attempts at chemotherapy.

Interested in mustard gas' newly-discovered capabilities of decimating white blood cells, two scientists by the names of Louis Goodman and Alfred Gilman tested its properties in the 1940s on mice. After administration of the gas, the regular white cells of the blood and the bone marrow had entirely disappeared. This success encouraged Gilman and Goodman to begin experimenting on humans, focusing on cancers of the lymph glands (lymphomas), organs comprised of white blood cells.

After treating a particular patient with ten continuous doses of mustard intravenously, the thoracic surgeon administering the treatment observed a remarkable remission of the patient's cancer. What followed, however, was a relapse of the tumor. Almost inevitably, the cancer had reappeared. As former director of the National Cancer Institute (NCI) Vincent DeVita once noted, "it took courage to be a chemotherapist [before] the 1960s and certainly the courage of the conviction that cancer would eventually succumb to drugs."

Before the 1980s, scientists had largely focused therapies on two fundamental vulnerabilities of cancer cells. Surgery and radiation therapy had exploited the fact that cancers originated as local diseases before spreading to secondary organs. These interventions attempted to eliminate cancer by physically excising the tumor before its cells had spread or by damaging cancer cells with localized administration of radiation. And early chemotherapies had exploited a second vulnerability – the rapid growth rate of particular cancer cells.

However, surgery and radiation therapy are inherently designed to be localized strategies; surgically removing multiple organs or tissues, or hitting various parts of the body with ionizing radiation would not be possible when cancer cells have spread beyond the primary organ or tissue, and especially if cancer cells have metastasized.

Cancer cells are driven to grow because of the inherent accumulation of DNA mutations - the activation of these proto-oncogenes and suppression of tumor-suppressor genes. The hallmarks of cancer - the ability to resist apoptotic signals, evade the immune system, metastasize to secondary organs, elicit the growth of new blood vessels, undergo atypical metabolic processes, and acquire advantageous mutations along the way - are derived from the corruption of correlating healthy physiological processes.

Identifying the subtle differences in these genes and acquired capabilities presented the central therapeutic question in the quest for the newest cancer medicines that followed. By the 1980s, the lab of Robert Weinberg had developed a technique to isolate cancer-causing genes (oncogenes) directly from cancer cells. The discovery of dozens of novel oncogenes had followed.

The Several Treatment Options for Cancer Patients

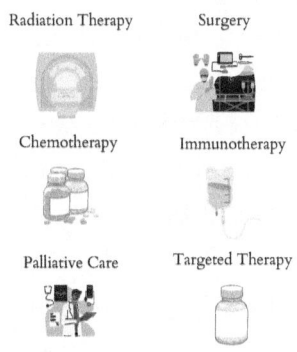

After years of research, another type of therapy had emerged that used drugs or chemical substances to precisely identify and target particular cellular receptors, antigens, molecules, or processes - known as *targeted therapy*.

There now exist more than 100 types of chemotherapy drugs, including alkylating agents, antimetabolites, antitumor antibiotics, and topoisomerase inhibitors, among others. This new, refined class of chemotherapeutic agents is the result of the search for drugs that target cells with high growth rates, impairing mitotic processes, and inducing cytotoxic effects on such cells. Topoisomerase inhibitors, for instance, are directed towards interfering with DNA replication in cancer cells (note that topoisomerase is the molecule that cleaves DNA strands during replicative processes to offer torsional-stress relief or to untangle replicating DNA).

The present chemotherapy regimen includes the administration of one or several chemotherapeutic agents, often used in combination with another intervention, including surgery, radiation, hormonal therapies, or other forms of cancer therapy. In addition to surgery and radiation therapy, cancers of the colon and kidneys are often treated with targeted therapies - EGFR inhibitors and VEGF inhibitors, molecules that inhibit the growth of new blood vessels and target angiogenesis. Likewise, various forms of skin cancer (melanoma) are often treated with BRAF inhibitors, and cancers of the liver are often treated with multikinase (Sorafenib). Cancers of the prostate are treated with anti-androgens.

Blood cancers, however, unlike solid tumors, often are treated with stem cell transplants, organ transplants, and tyrosine kinase inhibitors, such as Imatinib.

Through the sustained efforts in cancer drug discovery, once incurable forms of cancer, including Leukemia, Lymphoma, and tumors of the germline have been transformed into curable malignancies. Improved screening, refined diagnostic methods, and more effective treatment offerings have significantly improved the survival of cancer patients. Another class of significant contributors to the high survival rates now observed among cancer patients is the cohort of scientists and patients behind clinical studies for novel cancer drugs, including the studies controlled by the NSABP, MRC, EORTC, and the National Cancer Institute (NCI).

There has emerged yet another exciting development in the oncology field – immune therapy.

–

Immunotherapy

Cancer researchers have always had an eye on harnessing the capabilities of the immune system in the fight against tumors.

Immunotherapy (regarded as biological therapy) activates or suppresses the immune system to elicit (amplify) and or reduce (suppress) an immune response. Immunotherapy has captured great interest among researchers, clinicians, pharmaceutical corporations, and patients as well. However, scientists are presently unsure of the adverse effects of immunotherapy on the body.

Cell-based immunotherapies have shown great success in treating particular cancers. These therapies are designed to assist the effector cells of the immune system (lymphocytes, macrophages, dendritic cells, natural killer (NK) cells, and cytotoxic T lymphocytes) that typically work together to defend the body from cancer by targeting foreign antigens expressed on the surface of tumor cells.

The administration of a particular form of immunotherapy - Chimeric Antigen Receptor T-cell therapy (regarded as CAR T-cell Therapy) - has emerged as a growing practice in the treatment of cancer. This form of immunotherapy aims to assist in the production of T lymphocytes equipped to recognize and fight cancer cells in the body. T cells are extracted from the patient's blood and the gene responsible for producing particular -

antigen receptors are incorporated into the cells. These redeveloped T lymphocytes, each with CAR receptors on the cell surface, are further harvested and grown in vitro (in the lab), and infused back into the patient.

The basis for immunotherapies, similar to other interventions aimed at treating cancers, are purely scientific. It is the work of hundreds of thousands of scientists and years of ingenuity, persistence, and hopes for a better life for patients.

—

Generation after generation, we have increasingly prioritized the study of science and the practice of medicine. It has been this unwavering focus that has brought innovation in healthcare. Science has brought the most meaningful advances in our lives. As we explored through Elixir, it has been our deft understanding of our biology that has shaped our approach to medicine. The steadfast commitment to learning about our most intricate processes has yielded the greatest breakthroughs in human health.

EXPLORING LIFE

Author's Note

"The greatest need of humanity is the cure."

-Anonymous

In this book, we explored human life and disease. We explored our biochemistry and our molecular construct. We explored our genome, the instructions for our existence. We delved into our anatomy and physiology. We explored the circadian rhythm of our body, and its fascinating ubiquity throughout living systems around us. We explored the guardians of our well-being, our prized immunity. We delved into the maladies that have occluded our well-being for generations, as well as the mechanisms behind each disease. We explored the essence of curative medicine, delving into the discoveries and innovations that have advanced the medical field forward.

Where Malady represented disease, and Elixir represented cure, we delved into the relationship that has defined the medical field for centuries. Whether it be ancient Ayurvedic compounds or present-day stem cell therapies, our doctors and scientists have never stopped innovating.

Certain limits have been placed on what to include in this book, particularly in the interest of keeping it to a reasonable length. It would be mistaken to assume that each topic in this book has been given the thorough-most possible coverage. Having written this lengthy book at the age of sixteen, it is best to consider this my first version at an attempt to cover the most fascinating aspects of biology and medicine, a kind of handbook for the biomedical field.

—

All the doctors, scientists, physiologists, nurses, health practitioners, and advocates of science and medicine of our day, all the individuals on the front lines or behind the scenes; each of you have blessed humanity with the light that has kept and will continue to keep our world empowered.

It is clear that science has advanced medicine. That our fundamental understanding of our most intricate processes has offered us the greatest of insights. That the practice of research and discovery has yielded the greatest breakthroughs in healthcare. I hope this book has emphasized a crucial lesson:

Science has advanced medicine.

ACKNOWLEDGEMENTS

I would like to express heartfelt gratitude for the generosity, support, patience, love, insight, and wisdom of both my parents and my younger sister.

My utmost gratitude is further directed to the following individuals for supporting me, guiding me, and dedicating their precious time to my limitless curiosity throughout the creation of this book:

Dr. Nestor Ladron
Dr. Randy Schekman
Dr. William G. Kaelin
Dr. Mona Juneja
Dr. Sudip Parikh
Mr. Shawn Cyran
Dr. Brian Hall

SELECTED BIBLIOGRAPHY

Chaos

1. Reece, Jane B, and Neil A. Campbell. *Campbell Biology*. Boston: Benjamin C / Pearson, 2011. Print.
2. *"Protein Structure | Learn Science at Scitable."* Nature.com, 2014, www.nature.com/scitable/topicpage/protein-structure-14122136/.
3. *"Proteins and Gene Expression | Learn Science at Scitable."* Nature.com, 2014, www.nature.com/scitable/topic/proteins-and-gene-expression-14122688/.
4. Voet, Donald, et al. *Fundamentals of Biochemistry*. 5th ed., John Wiley & Sons, 2016.

Genome

1. Reece, Jane B, and Neil A. Campbell. *Campbell Biology*. Boston: Benjamin C / Pearson, 2011. Print.
2. *"Genomics and Medicine."* Genome.gov, 2019, www.genome.gov/health/Genomics-and-Medicine.
3. *"Talking Glossary of Genetic Terms | NHGRI."* Genome.gov, 2022, www.genome.gov/genetics-glossary.
4. *"What Is the Human Genome Project?"* Genome.gov, 2019, www.genome.gov/human-genome-project/What.
5. *"Human Genome Project Results."* Genome.gov, 2019, www.genome.gov/human-genome-project/results.
6. *"Human Genome Project FAQ."* Genome.gov, 2019, www.genome.gov/human-genome-project/Completion-FAQ.
7. *"Discoveries in Genetics."* Stanford.edu, 2022, web.stanford.edu/dept/news/stanfordtoday/ed/9611/9611fea1b01.shtml
8. Mendel, Gregor. *Discovery: Heredity Transmitted in Units.*

Facets

1. Reece, Jane B, and Neil A. Campbell. *Campbell Biology*. Boston: Benjamin C / Pearson, 2011. Print.
2. *"Your Digestive System & How It Works."* National Institute of Diabetes and Digestive and Kidney Diseases, NIDDK | National Institute of Diabetes and Digestive and Kidney Diseases.
3. *"How the Lungs Work - the Lungs | NHLBI, NIH."* Nih.gov, 24 Mar. 2022.
4. *"How the Lungs Work - the Respiratory System | NHLBI, NIH."* Nih.gov, 24 Mar. 2022, www.nhlbi.nih.gov/health/lungs/respiratory-system.
5. *"How the Lungs Work - What Breathing Does for the Body | NHLBI, NIH."* Nih.gov, 24 Mar. 2022
6. *"Microbiome."* National Institute of Environmental Health Sciences, 2018
7. Hiller-Sturmhöfel S, Bartke A. *The endocrine system: an overview.* Alcohol Health Res World. 1998;22(3):153-64. PMID: 15706790; PMCID: PMC6761896.
8. Nussey, Stephen, and Saffron Whitehead. *"Principles of Endocrinology."* Nih.gov, BIOS Scientific Publishers, 2022,
9. Tortora, Gerard J.,, and Bryan Derrickson. *Principles of Anatomy & Physiology.* 14th edition. Danvers, MA: Wiley, 2014. Print.

Rhythms

1. Reece, Jane B, and Neil A. Campbell. *Campbell Biology*. Boston: Benjamin C / Pearson, 2011. Print.
2. *"National Institute of General Medical Sciences (NIGMS) - Circadian Rhythms."* National Institute of General Medical Sciences (NIGMS), 2019.
3. *Circadian Rhythms and Circadian Clock*, 2022, www.cdc.gov/niosh/emres/longhourstraining/clock.html.
4. *"Michael W. Young - Our Scientists."* Our Scientists, 23 Dec. 2021, www.rockefeller.edu/our-scientists/heads-of-laboratories/914-michael-w-young/.

Immunity

1. Reece, Jane B, and Neil A. Campbell. *Campbell Biology*. Boston: Benjamin C / Pearson, 2011. Print.
2. Nicholson LB. *The immune system.* Biochem. 2016 Oct 31;60(3):275-301. doi: 10.1042/EBC20160017. PMID: 27784777; PMCID: PMC5091071.
3. *"Overview of the Immune System."* Nih.gov, 30 Dec. 2013, www.niaid.nih.gov/research/immune-system-overview.
4. *"Features of an Immune Response."* Nih.gov, 16 Jan. 2014, www.niaid.nih.gov/research/immune-response-features.
5. *"Immune Cells."* Nih.gov, 17 Jan. 2014, www.niaid.nih.gov/research/immune-cells.

Malady

1. Reece, Jane B, and Neil A. Campbell. *Campbell Biology*. Boston: Benjamin C / Pearson, 2011. Print.
2. *"Genetic Disorders."* Genome.gov, 2019, www.genome.gov/For-Patients-and-Families/Genetic-Disorders.
3. *"Disorders of the Immune System."* Nih.gov, 17 Jan. 2014, www.niaid.nih.gov/research/immune-system-disorders.
4. *"Immune Tolerance."* Nih.gov, 17 Jan. 2014, www.niaid.nih.gov/research/immune-tolerance.
5. *"Cancer."* National Institutes of Health (NIH), 28 Jan. 2020, www.nih.gov/about-nih/what-we-do/nih-turning-discovery-into-health/cancer-2020.
6. *"Understanding Cancer."* Nih.gov, National Institutes of Health (US), 2022, www.ncbi.nlm.nih.gov/books/NBK20362/.
7. *"What Is Cancer?"* National Cancer Institute, Cancer.gov, 5 May 2021, www.cancer.gov/about-cancer/understanding/what-is-cancer.
8. van Seventer, Jean Maguire, and Natasha S. Hochberg. "Principles of Infectious Diseases: Transmission, Diagnosis, Prevention, and Control." International Encyclopedia of Public Health, 2017, pp. 22–39

Elixir

1. *"Genomics and Medicine."* Genome.gov, 2019, www.genome.gov/health/Genomics-and-Medicine.
2. Reece, Jane B, and Neil A. Campbell. *Campbell Biology.* Boston: Benjamin C / Pearson, 2011. Print.
3. Isaacson, Walter, and Kathe Mazur. *The Code Breaker: Jennifer Doudna, Gene Editing, and the Future of the Human Race.* Print, 2021.
4. *"Stem Cell Basics | STEM Cell Information."* Nih.gov, 2016, stemcells.nih.gov/info/basics/stc-basics.
5. *"What Is Chemotherapy? | Chemo Treatment for Cancer."* Cancer.org, 2022, www.cancer.org/treatment/treatments-and-side-effects/treatment-types/chemotherapy.html.
6. *"Immunotherapy for Cancer."* National Cancer Institute, Cancer.gov, 24 Sept. 2019, www.cancer.gov/about-cancer/treatment/types/immunotherapy.
7. *"Ayurveda."* Hopkinsmedicine.org, 2 Dec. 2019, www.hopkinsmedicine.org/health/wellness-and-prevention/ayurveda.
8. *"Purpose of Surgery."* Hopkinsmedicine.org, 19 Nov. 2019, www.hopkinsmedicine.org/health/treatment-tests-and-therapies/purpose-of-having-surgery.
9. Pawson, Patricia, and Sandra Forsyth. *"Anesthetic Agents."* Small Animal Clinical Pharmacology, 2008, pp. 83–112
10. *"What Is Genetic Engineering?"* Yourgenome, 7 Oct. 2014

EXPANDED GLOSSARY

Acute: an occurrence that is sudden and does not last long

Adaptive immunity: type of immunity involving specialized immune cells and antibodies that target foreign antigens through memory of previous infections

Adenine: constituent base of nucleic acids, pairs with thymine in DNA and RNA

Adenosine triphosphate (ATP): energy currency of the cell, molecule

Adenosine: molecule found in cells, abundant in forms: adenosine, adenosine monophosphate (AMP), and adenosine triphosphate (ATP)

Adipose tissue: cells responsible for storing fatty acids as source of energy

Adrenal glands: endocrine glands next to the kidneys

Aerobic: capable of living, occurring, or existing only in an environment where oxygen is available

Allergen: any substance capable of inducing an allergic response in an individual

Allergy: damaging immune response by the body to a foreign substance resulting in hypersensitivity

Alpha cells: endocrine cells found in the Islets of Langerhans in the pancreas, secrete glucagon to increase glucose
levels in the blood stream

Alveoli: any air sac of the lung responsible for gaseous exchange (during breathing)

Alzheimer's disease: progressive disease resulting in loss of memory and neurodegeneration

Amnesia: loss of memories

Amygdala: region of gray matter inside each cerebral hemisphere, involved with experiencing of emotions

Amylase: enzyme responsible for digestion and hydrolysis of starch into simpler sugars

Anaerobic: capable of living, occurring, or existing in an environment where oxygen is unavailable

Analgesic: capable of relieving pain or sensations

EXPANDED GLOSSARY

Anemia: condition of low erythrocyte cell (red blood cell) count

Anesthesia: medical treatment used to prevent patients from feeling sensations during operational procedures, including surgery, dental work, and tissue sampling (biospy)

Anesthetic: any agent capable of inducing local or general loss of sensation or consciousness

Aneurysm: bulge in a blood vessel resulting from weakness in the blood vessel wall

Angiogenesis: production of new blood vessels

Angiotensin: peptide hormone resulting in vasoconstriction (constriction of blood vessels) and an increase in blood pressure

Antibiotic: a substance capable of inhibiting growth of microorganisms

Antibody: immunoglobulin, a blood protein produced and secreted in response to and counteracting a particular foreign antigen

EXPANDED GLOSSARY

Antigen-presenting cell: type of lymphocyte responsible for mediating the cellular immune response by processing and presenting antigens for recognition by T lymphocytes

Antigen: any toxin or foreign substance capable of inducing an immune response in the body, especially the production and secretion of antibodies (immunoglobulins)

Antihistamine: a class of drugs responsible for treating allergic conditions

Antioxidant: any substance capable of preventing or slowing damage to cells resulting from free radicals

Aorta: primary artery carrying blood away from the heart

Apoptosis: programmed cellular destruction

Arteriolosclerosis: thickening of the walls of the arterioles

Arteriosclerosis: thickening of the walls of the arteries

Artery: blood vessel carrying mostly-oxygenated blood away from the heart to all parts of the body

EXPANDED GLOSSARY

Arthritis: swelling and tenderness of one or more joints

Asthma: narrowing of the airways in the lungs

Atherosclerosis: deposition of cholesterol plaques and fatty acids in the walls of the artery

Atrium: one of two upper chambers in the heart receiving blood from circulation

Auditory nerve: either of the eight pair of cranial nerves connecting the inner ear with the brain

Autoimmunity: condition when the body's immune system is unable to differentiate between one's own cells and foreign cells

Autonomic nervous system: component of the peripheral nervous system regulating involuntary physiological processes, including heartbeat, blood pressure, respiration, and digestion

B cell: lymphocyte responsible for humoral immunity in the adaptive immune system, capable of producinge
antibodies (immunoglobulin)

Bacterium: a unicellular microorganism lacking organlles and a nucleus, oftentimes pathogenic

EXPANDED GLOSSARY

Benign tumor: uncontrolled cell growth that does not appear to be cancerous

Beta cells: endocrine cells found in the Islets of Langerhans in the pancreas, secrete insulin to control the level of glucose in the bloodstream

Bile: alkaline fluid that aids digestion and is secreted by the liver

Bioavailability: proportion of a drug or substance that enters the circulation when introduced into the body, capable of inducing an active effect

Biomarker: biological molecule found in blood or tissues that is a sign of occurence of a given process, condition, or disease

Biopsy: sampling of an organ's tissue for examination

Blood pressure: the pressure of circulating blood against the walls of blood vessels

Blood vessel: passageway facilitating the circulation of blood throughout the body, including arteries, arterioles, veins, venules, and capillaries

Body mass index: value derived from the mass and height of a person

EXPANDED GLOSSARY

Brain stem: region of brain connected to the spinal cord, regulating breathing and heart rhythms

Bronchiole: branch where bronchus divides into within the lungs

Caffeine: natural substance with stimulant effects including cognitive enhancement and increased alertness, inhibits binding of adenosine to receptors in the brain

Calcitonin: hormone produced by the thyroid responsible for regulating the use of calcium in the body

Calcium: compound responsible for healthy blood clotting, contactility, heart rhythms, neuronal synapses, and structural support for bones and teeth

Cancer: condition of malignant growth of cells

Capillary: branching blood vessel forming a network between the arterioles and venules

Carbohydrate: biomolecule consisting of carbon, hydrogen, and oxygen atoms, responsible for providing energy for metabolism in the cell

Carcinogen: any agent or substance capable of inducing cancer in an organism

Cardiovascular: pertaining to the blood flow and blood vessels in the heart

EXPANDED GLOSSARY

Cell: smallest living structural and functional unit of a living organism

Cerebellum: structure located behind the brain responsible for coordination of movement and balance

Cerebral cortex: outermost layer of the brain associated with highest mental capabilities

Cerebrovascular: pertaining to blood flow or the blood vessels in the brain

Chemotherapy: type of treatment offering chemicals and anti-cancer drugs to target fast-growing cells as a part of a standardized chemotherapy regimen

Cholesterol: lipid substance and organic biosynthesized by all animal cells and an essential structural component of animal cell membranes

Chromosome: threadlike structure of nucleic acids and protein found in the nucleus of living cells, carries genetic information through genes

Chronic: an occurrence that is gradual and remains for a lengthy period of time

EXPANDED GLOSSARY

Chyme: the pulpy acidic fluid transported from the stomach to the small intestine

Circadian rhythm: natural, internal process regulating the sleep-wake cycle and repeating every 24 hours

Collagen: fiber-like protein found in connective tissue, responsible for providing structural support in organs and tissues

Congestion: swelling of nasal passages with excess fluid and mucus

Connective tissue: tissue supporting, protecting, and giving structure to nearby tissues and organs in the body

Cornea: the clear, protective outer layer of the eye

Coronary artery: artery responsible for supplying blood to the heart

Cortisol: primary hormone for inducing stress, responsible for increased glucose cencentrations in the bloodstream

Cytokine: a substance (interferon, interleukin, growth factors) secreted through cells of the immune system

EXPANDED GLOSSARY

Cytosine: constituent base of nucleic acids, pairs with guanine in DNA

Dendrite: appendages designed to receive communications from nearby cells

Dendritic cell: professional antigen-presenting cells essential for the induction of protective immune responses against pathogens

Dentin: part of the tooth beneath the enamel and cementum

Diabetes: chronic health condition affecting the body's ability to metabolize glucose

DNA: organic chemical containing genetic information and the instructions required for protein synthesis

Enamel: outer covering of the tooth

Enteropathy: any disease or swelling of the small intestine

Eosinophil: white blood cells with large granules responsible for targeting infections

Epidemic: widespread occurrence of an infectious disease in a particular community

EXPANDED GLOSSARY

Epinephrine: hormone and neurotransmitter responsible for regulating visceral functions, including heart rates, contractility of heart, rate of respiration, glycogenolysis in the liver, and vasoconstriction and vasodilation

Epithelial cell: cell responsible for lining the surfaces of the body

Epithelium: tissue forming the outer layer of body's surface and outer lining of hollow structures and organs

Esophagus: hollow passageway carrying food and liquid to the stomach

Fatigue: feeling of constant weakness

Fiber: type of carbohydrate ingestible for the body's digestive enzymes

Fibroblast: type of biological cell responsible for synthesizing the extracellular matrix and collagen

Flavonoids: class of polyphenolic metabolites found in plants, responsible for vivid colors in fruits and vegetables with carotenoids

Floaters: spots in vision that resemble black or light strings that drift across the eyes

EXPANDED GLOSSARY

Free radical: any species of molecule capable of independent existence containing an unpaired electron in atomic orbit, unstable atoms

Fructose: type of monosaccharide sugar naturally occurring in fruits

Fungi: spore-producing organisms including molds, yeast, mushrooms

Ganglion: group of neurons in the PNS

Gastrointestinal tract: series of hollow organs responsible for the ingestion, digestion, and absorption of nutrients

Gene: a unit of heredity transferred from parent to offspring, a distinct seuqnece of nucleotides

Genetic: pertaining to genes or hereditary

Ghrelin: a hormone produced to increase appetite

Gland: an organ responsible for secreting particular hormones

EXPANDED GLOSSARY

Glial cell: non-neuronal cells located in the CNS and PNS, responsible for providing metabolic support ot neurons, including neuronal insulation, communication, and transport of nutrients.

Glioblastoma: fast-growing, aggressive tumor of the brain

Glioma: a type of tumor occurring in the brain and spinal cord

Glucagon: hormone produced by alpha cells of the pancreas to regulate glucose levels in the plasma and release of
glucose into circulation

Glucose: main monosaccharide found in our bloodstream, simply sugar with the molecular formula $C_6H_{12}O_6$

Glutamate: excitatory neurotransmitter released by neurons in the brain

Glycogen: multibranched polysaccharide of glucose, serves as a form of energy storage in organisms

Growth factor: substance capable of stimulating cell proliferation and cellular differentiation

EXPANDED GLOSSARY

Guanine: constituent base of nucleic acids, pairs with cytosine in DNA and uracil in RNA

Hemoglobin: protein found in red blood cells (erythrocytes) responsible for carrying oxygen

High blood pressure: condition involving higher than usual force of blood against the walls of the artery (hypertension)

Hippocampus: component of the brain involved in consolidation of information to long-term memory

Histamine: inflammatory compound released by cells during an allergic or inflammatory reaction, results in the contraction of smooth muscle tissue and dilation of capillaries

Homeostasis: state of steady internal physiological and chemical conditions maintained by living systems

Hormone: signaling molecule transported to distant or nearby organs to regulate physiology

Hyperglycemia: high blood glucose

Hyperthyroidism: excess production of thyroxine hormone by the thyroid gland

Hypoglycemia: low blood glucose

EXPANDED GLOSSARY

Hypoglycemia: low blood glucose

Hypothalamus: region of the brain below the thalamus, responsible for coordinating both autonomic nervous
system and activity of the pituitary gland (controlling body temperature, thirst, hunger, homeostasis, sleep, etc.)

Hypoxia: condition of less oxygen

Immunization: process where an individual develops immunity towards a particular disease through vaccination or inoculation

Immunoglobulin: antibody, glycoprotein molecule produced by white blood cells responsible for binding to antigens

Immunosuppressant: any agent capable of suppressing the immune system

Immunotherapy: type of treatment offering activation or suppression of the immune system

Infection: invasion or growth germs in the body

Innate immunity: type of immunity involving the first line of defense against pathogens, phagocytic barriers, non-specific cytokines

EXPANDED GLOSSARY

Insulin: hormone produced by beta cells of the pancreas, regulates the metabolism of carbohydrates

Interleukin: protein produced by leukocytes (white blood cells) responsible for regulating immune response

Keratin: a protein and major component of the cuticle and cortex layers of the hair

Keratinocytes: cells that produce keratin protein

Ketone: substance produced when the body begins to burn adipose tissue for energy

Lactase: enzyme that breaks down milk sugar (lactose)

Lactose intolerance: inability of the body to digest lactose sugars

Langerhans cells: cells of the immune system found in the skin

Leptin: a hormone produced by adipose tissue to suppress appetite and burn stored lipids

Leukocyte: white blood cell (granulocytes, monocytes, lymphocytes)

Leukotrienes: chemicals that result in swelling of the airways when an allergic reaction occurs or in diseases like asthma

Levothyroxine sodium: an artificially-produced form of the thyroid hormone thyroxine

Lipase: an enzyme secreted by the pancreas to help the body break down lipids

Lipid: a class of organic compounds that are fatty acids or derivatives of fatty acids, insoluble in water and soluble in organic solvents

Lipid: fats, oils, and waxes that serve as the building blocks for cells or as energy sources

Lipoprotein: a combination of lipid and protein molecules bound together, allowing for convenient circulation
through blood

Liver: vital organ that removes toxic waste products from the body and helps in digestion

Lymph nodes: small organs that filter germs and pathogens out of the body

Lymphocyte: a type of white blood cell with the ability to recognize foreign substances in the body

EXPANDED GLOSSARY

Magnetic resonance imaging (MRI): scan that creates pictures of internal organs using radio waves, strong magnetic fields, and computing power

Major Histocompatibility Complex Molecule (MHC): molecule that helps protect the body from foreign substances with cell-surface proteins

Malignant Tumor: cancerous growth of cells

Mast cell: cell involved in allergic reactions, and when stimulated, releases chemicals (i.e. histamine) that signal infection and activate an inflammatory response

Melanin: a protein and major component of skin colors

Melanocytes: cells that produce melanin protein

Melatonin: hormone released by the pineal gland of the brain, associated with the sleep-wake cycle

Microbe: any microorganism

Mitochondrion: small cellular structures that break down glucose sugars into energy (ATP)

Monoclonal antibody: artificially-produced antibody used to treat certain diseases

EXPANDED GLOSSARY

Monocytes: white blood cells (leukocytes) that protect the body from disease by attacking and consuming foreign particles

Motilin: hormone that facilitates the contraction of the small intestine and the motion of food through the digestive tract.

Mucous membrane: a thin layer lining many cavities and structures in the body that are exposed to air in the environment, including the nose, mouth, and lungs

Mutation: a particular alteration in the genetic sequence of an organism

Nebulizer: device that converts a liquid medicine into a breathable mist

Necrosis: the premature death of living cells or tissues

Neoplasm: an abnormal growth of tissue, either benign or malignant

Nerve growth factor: molecule that promotes the growth and repair of nerve cells

Neurodegeneration: progressive atrophy and loss of function of neurons in the brain

EXPANDED GLOSSARY

Neuron: fundamental cellular unit of the brain and nervous system

Neurotransmitter: a chemical messenger released by neurons that transmits messages to nearby neurons through a synapse

Nociceptors: nerve endings that detect pain and transmit pain information to the brain and spinal cord for recognition

Non-REM Sleep: phase of the sleep cycle that includes deep sleep

Norepinephrine: hormone produced by adrenal glands that keep the body on heightened alert when a threat is perceived, alternatively known as noradrenaline

Nucleic acid: large biomolecules responsible for the storage and expression of genetic information

Nutrient: substances that the body requires to survive, often obtain through ingestion and inhalation

Oncogene: a gene whose expression, under particular conditions, may cause cancer

Oxidant: an unstable molecule in the body, plays a role in aging and may damage tissue, free radical

EXPANDED GLOSSARY

Oxidation: a process where oxygen combines with a substance, altering its structure, form, and function.

Pancreas: gland that produce digestive enzymes and hormones

Pandemic: a disease outbreak affecting large populations or a whole region

Protein: large biomolecules comprised of long chains of amino acids and polypeptides, forms include enzymes, hormones, growth factors, transport proteins, structural proteins

Radiation therapy: type of treatment offering ionizing radiation to destroy malignant cells and typically delivered by a linear accelerator

Rapid Eye Movement (REM) Sleep: phase of the sleep cycle that includes rapid movements of the eye and vivid dreaming during sleep

Senescence: the condition or process of deterioration with age or the progressive loss of a cell's ability to grow and proliferate

Surgery: medical procedure using instrumental techniques on a patient to investigate or treat a pathological condition

EXPANDED GLOSSARY

Synapse: the site of transmittance of electric or chemical signals between neurons

Thalamus: large mass of gray matter located in the dorsal part of the brain, serves in relaying of sensory signals to the cerebral cortex and regulation of consciousness, sleep, and alertness.

Thymine: constituent base of nucleic acids, pairs with adenine in DNA and RNA

ABOUT THE AUTHOR

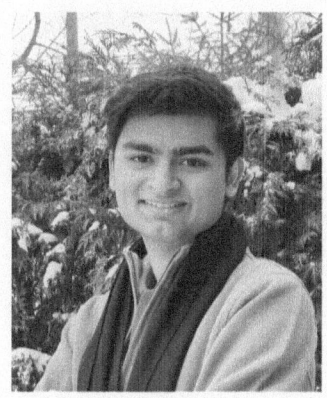

The author of *Exploring Life: Probing Human Life & Disease*, Param is a science researcher, journalist, and an avid, lifelong student of medicine. Param founded and currently serves as Editor-in-Chief of Academy SciJournal, the premier scientific publication of the Academies at Englewood, where he has interviewed several distinguished scientific leaders and published dozens of articles and studies. He has authored several academic publications regarding his research on brain cancers, particularly on *Glioblastoma Multiforme* (GBM).

Param is additionally a member of the American Association of Cancer Research (AACR), the New Jersey Academy of Science (NJAS), the Academy Medical Society (AMS), and the American Red Cross. A driven, life-long student of the biomedical sciences, Param lives near New York City and aspires to impact the world through science, innovation, and discovery.

www.ingramcontent.com/pod-product-compliance
Lightning Source LLC
Chambersburg PA
CBHW031620210526
45464CB00004B/1666